THE INTELLIGENT PATIENT GUIDE TO
COLORECTAL CANCER

Other books in the Intelligent Patient Guide series include:

The Intelligent Patient Guide to
Breast Cancer, 3rd edition
by Ivo Olivotto, MD, Karen Gelmon, MD, Urve Kuusk, MD
ISBN 0-9696125-6-7

The Intelligent Patient Guide to
Prostate Cancer, 3rd edition
by S. Larry Goldenberg, MD, Ian M. Thompson, MD
ISBN 0-9696125-5-9

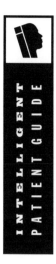

INTELLIGENT PATIENT GUIDE

THE INTELLIGENT PATIENT GUIDE TO

COLORECTAL CANCER

ALL YOU NEED TO KNOW TO TAKE AN ACTIVE PART IN YOUR TREATMENT

MICHAEL E. PEZIM MD FRCSC FACS
DAVID A. OWEN MB FRCPath FRCPC

EDITOR
JAY DRAPER
CONTRIBUTING EDITOR
CHERYL EDWARDS MA

SECOND EDITION, VANCOUVER, BC 2005

While the authors have made every effort to ensure that the material contained herein is accurate at time of publication, new discoveries or changes in treatment practices may ultimately invalidate some of the information presented here.

To obtain a copy of this guide, or others in the series, write:
Intelligent Patient Guide Ltd. Suite 30, 3195 Granville St.,
Vancouver, BC, Canada V6H 3K2
www.ipguide.com
email: info@ipguide.com

Copyright ©2005 by Intelligent Patient Guide Ltd.

Library and Archives Canada Cataloguing In Publication

Pezim, Michael E. (Michael Elliot), 1953–
The intelligent patient guide to colorectal cancer / Michael E. Pezim, David Owen—2nd ed.

(Intelligent Patient Guide)
Includes index.
Previous ed., by Michael E. Pezim, published 1992 under title:
The intelligent patient guide to colon & rectal cancer.
ISBN 0-9696125-7-5

1. Colon (Anatomy)—Cancer—Popular works. 2. Rectum—Cancer—Popular works.
I. Owen, David A. II. Pezim, Michael E. (Michael Elliot), 1953– .
Intelligent patient guide to colon & rectal cancer. III. Title. IV. Title: Colorectal cancer. V. Series.
RC280.C6P49 2005   616.99'4347   C2005-903109-3

Printed in Canada

AUTHORS

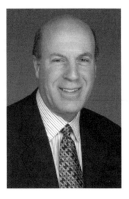

Michael E. Pezim, MD FRCSC FACS

Dr. Pezim is the Medical Director of the Pezim Clinic, an intestinal diagnostic and treatment center in Vancouver. He received his MD from the University of Toronto and surgical training at the University of British Columbia. He was a surgical fellow in colon and rectal surgery at the Mayo Clinic. Prior to entering private practice, Dr. Pezim was an Associate Professor of Surgery and Head of the Section of Colon and Rectal Surgery at the University of British Columbia and a Consultant to the BC Cancer Agency.

David A. Owen, MB FRCPath FRCPC

Dr. Owen is a Professor of Pathology at the University of British Columbia and a consultant pathologist at Vancouver General Hospital and the BC Cancer Agency. He received his medical and pathology training at St. Thomas' Hospital Medical School in London, England. Dr. Owen has long been a favorite teacher of pathologists-in-training and is regarded as one of the most capable gastrointestinal pathologists in North America.

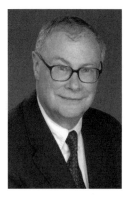

EDITOR
Jay Draper

CONTRIBUTING EDITOR
Cheryl Edwards, MA

COORDINATOR
Nicola Sutton, BA MBA

ILLUSTRATORS
Vicky Earle
Peter Woods

DESIGN
MURPHYWOODS Creative & Design

GRAPHIC PRODUCTION
Angela G. Atkins

CONTRIBUTING AUTHORS

Jacqueline A. Brown, BScN MD FRCPC
Assistant Professor, Department of
Radiology, University of British Columbia
Staff Radiologist, St. Paul's Hospital,
Vancouver, BC

Bruce B. Forster, MD FRCP
Associate Professor, Department of
Radiology, University of British Columbia
Medical Director, Canada Diagnostic Centres
Vancouver, BC

Dianne E. Garde, ET
Enterostomal Therapy Advisor, Ostomy
Association, Toronto, ON
Canadian Society for Enterostomal Therapy
World Council of Enterostomal Therapists

John Hay, MD FRCPC
Radiation Oncologist, BC Cancer Agency

Shirley Hobenshield, RDN
Registered Dietician-Nutritionist
BC Cancer Agency

Doug Horsman, MD FCRP FCCMG
Clinical Professor, Department of Pathology
and Laboratory Medicine, University of
British Columbia
Director, Hereditary Cancer Program,
BC Cancer Agency

Kathleen Kaulback
Clinical Psychologist

Mary McCullum, RN MSN CON(C)
Nurse Educator, Hereditary Cancer Program
BC Cancer Agency

Robin O'Brien, Pharm D BCOP
Oncology Pharmacist
BC Cancer Agency

Cathy Rayment
Provincial Library Leader
BC Cancer Agency

Amil Shah, MD FRCPC
Medical Oncologist, BC Cancer Agency

Cheri Van Patten, MSc RDN
Registered Dietician Nutritionist
BC Cancer Agency

This book is dedicated to our patients whose courage, dignity and quest for answers have inspired us.

We would also like to acknowledge those who most encouraged us to become physicians with two personal dedications:

Dr. Michael Pezim dedicates his work to Bernice Pezim.

Dr. David Owen dedicates his work to Daniel Owen.

CONTENTS

(continued)

CONTENTS *(continued)*

WHY READ THIS BOOK?

When cancer crosses the threshold of your life, it is as if your world has shattered. Like so many others, you look for ways to summon the strength needed to face your greatest challenge ever. No one would choose this challenge, but every cancer patient is given a choice—the choice of *how* to face the unwanted journey.

Most people find strength from within, from loved ones, their faith, skillful medical teams, and from what they learn along the way. And, amazingly, many of the survivors say their experience with cancer made them look at life differently and, after recovery, they made changes that enriched their lives.

Still, when you are undergoing cancer treatment, the feeling that you've lost control of your life brings deep despair. What is to be done to help you regain control? Not only does the answer lie within the pages of this book, but the very act of reading a book about your cancer is an important step towards self-empowerment. The expression, "knowledge is power" is what *The Intelligent Patient Guide Series* is all about. A series of books that offer you the most accurate medical information delivered in a style tailored for a layperson is a profound source of comfort and practical usefulness.

Understanding your disease more fully while learning about choices and reasons for specific treatments is crucial. Strategies for coping, common emotional responses, ways to handle side effects, finding out what to expect—all this information helps you take charge.

Although doctors and medical staff will inform you of your treatment choices and the nature of your case, their time is in high demand. That is why a book that provides a more complete picture is needed. As you read this book and learn more about your disease, your doctor will be able to offer you more because you will know what questions to ask. And you will understand the answers more fully.

We have created this book to provide you with the very best information in the hope that you will make the strong choice. You will choose to be informed about what most concerns you using the knowledge and advice in these pages. You will choose courage and hope. Though the journey was unwanted, you will choose the way you face the future and your inner spirit will prevail.

Cheryl Edwards, MA
Contributing Editor

ONE

COLORECTAL CANCER:
WHAT IS IT AND HOW IS IT DETECTED?

1

WHAT IS CANCER?

To understand what cancer is, it is important to know a few basic principles of how body cells normally behave.

NORMAL CELL GROWTH AND CANCER

The body is made up of tiny cells, for example, skin cells, muscle cells, heart cells, nerve cells, and bone cells. When a baby grows, the number of cells increases very quickly. A cell becomes a bit larger, and then divides into two new cells (Figure 1). After a period of time, each of these cells divides again, and so on. Once a child grows to adulthood, the size of the body no longer increases. However, our bodies go through a lot of wear and tear, both inside and outside. Worn-out cells constantly need to be replaced, so cell division still continues, but more slowly. One visible change is the tiny bits of dead skin flaking off as the skin constantly renews itself.

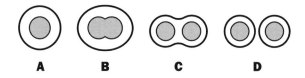

Figure 1. *Normal cell division. A cell grows a bit larger and then divides into two cells.*

Although an adult's cells continue to divide, it happens in an orderly, controlled way. This is because each cell carries genetic instructions that regulate how fast the cell should divide and grow and when the cell should die. A balance between cells growing and dying keeps our bodies functioning normally.

WHEN CELL GROWTH GOES OUT OF CONTROL

Sometimes a cell starts to grow without regard for the normal balance between cell growth and death, and a small, harmless lump of cells will form. These harmless growths are referred to as *benign*. A benign growth can occur in any part of the body, including the breast, skin, or intestines.

In other cases, a cell may grow and divide with complete disregard for the needs and limitations of the body. These cells have the potential to grow into large masses or spread to other areas of the body. Cells that have this aggressive behavior are called *malignant*. A mass of such cells is called a *cancer*. When clumps of these cells spread to other parts of the body and begin growing there as cancer spots, they are called *metastases*. A cancer that continues to grow can eventually overwhelm and destroy the part of the body or particular organ where it is located.

CANCER CELLS HAVE THE ABILITY TO SPREAD

Normal cells remain in the area where they belong and don't spread to other parts of the body. Cancer cells, on the other hand, spread through the body in three ways (Figure 2). They could grow directly into a neighboring organ or

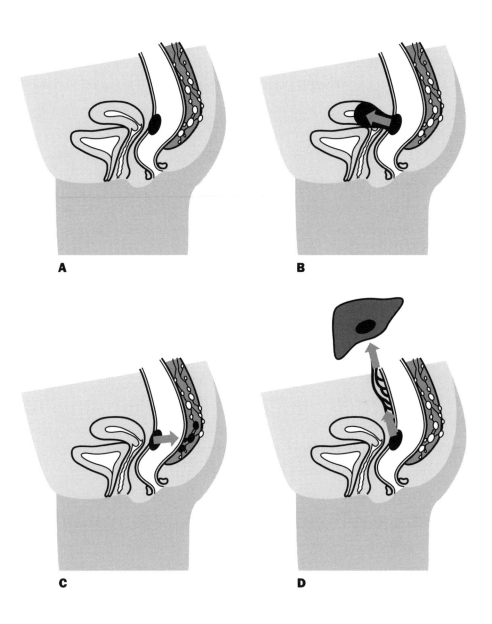

Figure 2. *Cancer spread. Cancer (A) grows and spreads by direct local invasion (B), or to lymph nodes (C), or through the blood stream to far-away organs such as the liver, lungs, or brain (D).*

spread through the blood stream to far-away organs such as the lungs, liver, and bones. They can also spread into the lymph nodes.

When a cancer spreads, it still retains the properties of the original cancer. This means that a colon cancer that spreads to the liver is still a colon cancer. Under the microscope, it looks just like a colon cancer. Its cells do not look like liver cells or liver cancer cells, and it responds to treatment like a colon cancer, not a liver cancer. Doctors refer to the original cancer in the colon as the *primary cancer*. Cancer spots that have originated from the primary cancer are called *secondary cancer* or *metastatic cancer*. Thus, a colon cancer patient with metastases in the liver might be referred to by a physician as having a colon cancer primary with so-called secondaries in the liver.

CANCER CELLS CAN TRICK THE IMMUNE SYSTEM

The immune system consists of a group of cells called white blood cells, which recognize and destroy foreign material in the body such as bacteria, viruses, and unfamiliar or abnormal cells. Cancer cells somehow manage to avoid being stopped by the immune system.

COLORECTAL CANCER DOES NOT DEVELOP OVERNIGHT

It can take years of cell division before a normal cell becomes a cancerous cell. The cell first undergoes very small changes in which it becomes slightly abnormal. It may also begin to divide, grow more quickly, and accumulate in excessive numbers. At some point, the collection of abnormal cells becomes visible to the naked eye as a lump. If this occurs on the lining of the colon or rectum, it is called a *polyp*. Polyps may remain benign (abnormal but not cancerous) or become even more abnormal-looking, and finally turn cancerous (Figure 3).

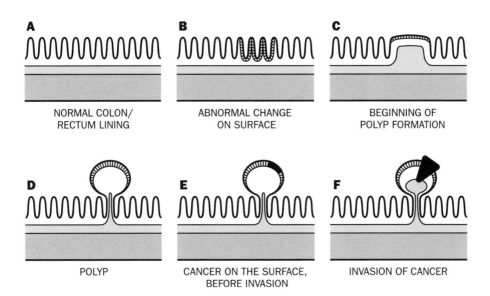

Figure 3. *Cancer development. Colon cancer does not develop overnight. Gradually the cells become more and more abnormal until, eventually, they become cancer cells. Cancer cells are initially confined to the surface. Later, they can grow deeper and become invasive colorectal cancer cells.*

THE COLON AND RECTUM IN
HEALTH AND DISEASE

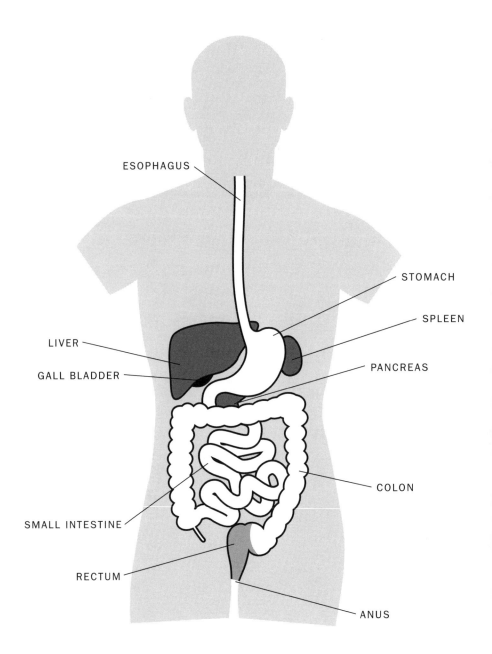

Figure 4. *The gastrointestinal (GI) tract.*

CHAPTER 2
ANATOMY AND FUNCTION OF
THE COLON AND RECTUM

AN OVERVIEW OF THE GASTROINTESTINAL TRACT

The gastrointestinal (GI) tract is a long passage that begins at the mouth and ends at the anus (Figure 4). Its purpose is to transport food through a process of digestion, absorption, and elimination.

In the upper GI tract, the teeth begin the process of digestion by grinding food into small fragments that the esophagus then pushes down to the stomach. Here, strong acid liquefies the food, which is then delivered, in spurts, into the duodenum to be mixed with bile from the liver and enzymes from the pancreas. This mixture then travels through the seven meters (23 feet) of small intestine where the tiny food particles are absorbed into the bloodstream and taken to the liver. Finally, the liver transforms the food particles into molecules that give energy to the body.

By the time the mixture has passed through the full length of the small intestine, most of its nutritional value has been absorbed into the bloodstream, leaving a watery green waste product. This travels into the large intestine, also called the *colon*, where the remaining fluid is absorbed, and the material is compacted, stored, and ultimately expelled.

THE COLON AND RECTUM

Much like a square picture frame, the colon sits like a large square within the abdomen. It begins in the lower right side of the abdomen, travels up, then turns across the midline and descends the left side of the abdomen (Figure 5).

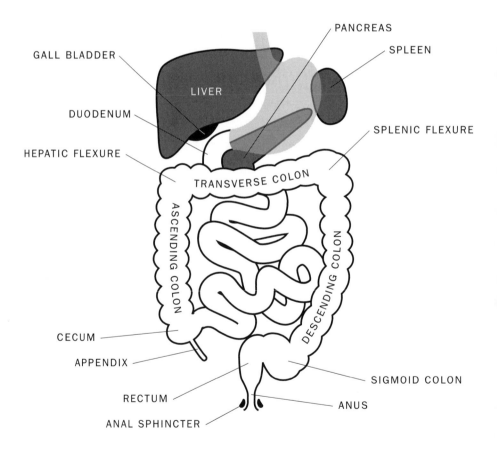

Figure 5. *The colon (large intestine).*

This is the path that food takes after it leaves the small intestine. It first enters the colon through the *cecum*, then goes up the *ascending colon*, across the *transverse colon*, and down the *descending colon*. The descending colon ends with the s-shaped *sigmoid colon*, and finally the *rectum*. The rectum, lying within the protection of the pelvic bones, forms the last 15 cm (seven inches) of the colon. The last three cm (one inch) of the rectum is the anus with its encircling sphincter muscles.

THE UNIQUE BLOOD DRAINAGE SYSTEM
OF THE COLON AND RECTUM

Blood from most of the body's organs drains directly back to the heart for re-circulation. However, because the liver is so important in the digestive system,* the blood that contains the absorbed food particles from the large and small intestine travels directly to the liver, through a special system of veins, without first going to any other part of the body. This special system of veins is called the portal venous system (Figure 6).

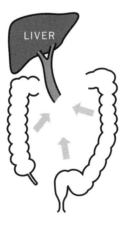

Figure 6. *Blood from the colon flows directly to the liver.*

---

* The body can't really use food particles until they have been modified by the liver.

The portal venous system plays a special role in colorectal cancer. Sometimes, small clumps of cancer cells from a colorectal cancer will break off from the main body of a cancer and drift within the blood and food particles of the portal venous system to the liver. Here, they implant and grow into tumor masses, called *liver metastases*. When colorectal cancer spreads, two-thirds of the time, it spreads to the liver.

LYMPHATIC DRAINAGE OF THE COLON AND RECTUM

Most people understand that our bodies contain arteries and veins to transport blood, but few people are aware that there is another system of vessels in the body. It is called the *lymphatic system* and its job is to collect fluid that would otherwise accumulate in our tissues. This fluid, referred to as *lymph*, is channeled away by a network of tiny tubes that are mostly invisible to the naked eye called *lymphatic vessels*. The lymphatic vessels direct the lymph toward larger lymphatic vessels in the center of the abdomen and then upward into the back of the chest cavity. From there, the lymphatic vessels connect to a large vein behind the left collarbone where the lymph flows into the bloodstream (Figure 7).

In addition to draining away fluid, the lymphatic system plays an important role in fighting infection. Spaced along the lymphatic vessels are groups of lima bean shaped structures, *lymph nodes*, where infection-fighting antibodies are produced to combat bacteria, viruses, and abnormal cells floating in the lymph.

Just as the blood vessels provide a pathway for cancer cells to spread to faraway organs, the lymphatic vessels provide cancer cells with a way of spreading into lymph nodes. Once in a lymph node, cancer cells may implant and begin to grow. A growing group of cancer cells within a lymph node is called a *lymph node metastasis*. When a colon or rectal cancer is removed, a physician who specializes in examining diseased tissue, a *pathologist*, will examine

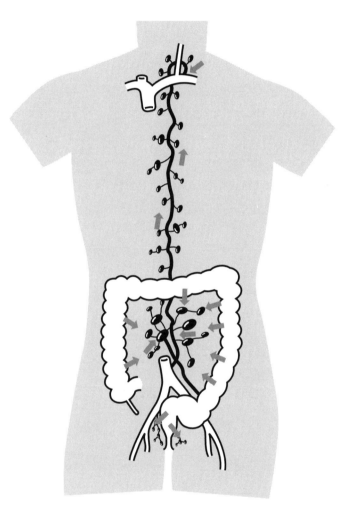

Figure 7. *The lymphatic drainage system of the colon and rectum.*

each lymph node in the specimen to see whether it contains cancer. The finding of cancer in the lymph nodes will have an impact on whether additional treatment, such as chemotherapy, should be given following surgery.

SPECIAL LYMPH NODE ANATOMY OF THE RECTUM

The lymph nodes of the rectum lie in a collection of fat attached to the back of the rectum called the *mesorectum*. The rectum and mesorectum are contained by a membrane, the *mesorectal fascia*, that separates them from the rest of the pelvic tissues (Figure 8). When operating on rectal cancer, the surgeon maximizes the patient's chance for cure by removing the rectum, mesorectum, and encircling mesorectal fascia in one piece so the lymph nodes and any cancer cells they could contain remain undisturbed.

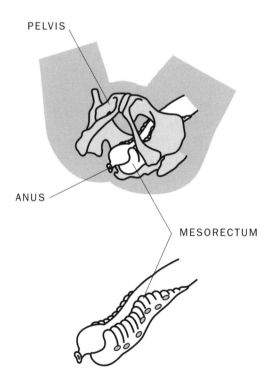

Figure 8a. *The mesorectum surrounds the back and sides of the rectum.*

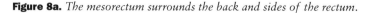

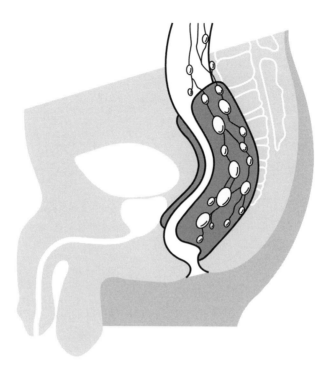

Figure 8b. *Side view of the mesorectum.*

CHAPTER 3

DISORDERS OF THE COLON AND RECTUM
THAT MAY BE CONFUSED WITH CANCER

The colon and rectum are susceptible to a number of non-cancerous disorders. Sometimes these disorders cause symptoms that are similar to those of cancer, so careful examination and diagnostic testing may be required to distinguish the true nature of the patient's condition.

APPENDICITIS

The appendix is attached to the bottom of the cecum, in the right lower side of the abdomen. Sometimes stool or swelling will block the opening of the appendix. The blocked appendix becomes inflamed (known as *appendicitis*). If the blockage does not go away, the appendix may rupture.

DIVERTICULITIS

With aging, the colon may develop small outpouchings of its walls. These are called *diverticula* (plural of diverticulum). Diverticula are thought to be due to localized areas of high pressure resulting from intestinal spasm. The condition of multiple diverticula is known as *diverticulosis*. Diverticulosis is very common. In certain populations, 40% of individuals over the age of 50 will have diverticulosis. On rare occasions, a diverticulum can burst, leading to inflammation known as *diverticulitis*. Diverticula occur most often in the sigmoid colon, so diverticulitis usually causes pain in the lower left side of the abdomen, and is generally associated with fever and pain. It is thought that the high pressure spasms that lead to diverticulosis are partly due to low intake of dietary fiber, since diverticulosis is seen most commonly in Western countries where much of the diet consists of highly refined carbohydrates. However, the true cause of diverticula remains unknown.

IRRITABLE BOWEL SYNDROME

The walls of the colon are muscular. Colon muscle may develop frequent spasms or coordination problems, which can create a condition called *irritable bowel syndrome (IBS)*. IBS is characterized by alternating bouts of diarrhea and constipation, abdominal cramping, bloating, and frequent urgent bowel movements shortly after eating. It is diagnosed by first eliminating the possibility of more serious causes of these symptoms. Although IBS is not serious, it can be a very distressing condition.

INFLAMMATORY BOWEL DISEASE

The colon and rectum are susceptible to developing inflammation called *inflammatory bowel disease (IBD)*. There are two characteristic patterns of inflammation; one called *ulcerative colitis* and the other named *Crohn's disease*. These diseases are treated with anti-inflammatory medications and sometimes surgery if they are severe and unresponsive to non-surgical treatments.

VASCULAR DISEASES OF THE COLON

Aging and abnormal thickening of the arteries (accelerated by smoking, high blood pressure, diabetes, etc.) can lead to blockage of the blood vessels that supply the colon. If a blood vessel blocks suddenly, the colon can become swollen and painful, and may ooze dark blood. This condition is called *ischemic colitis* and is usually seen in elderly patients with other cardiovascular conditions. The early symptoms of pain and colon blockage may be difficult to distinguish from diverticulitis, since both conditions usually occur in the left side of the colon.

HEMORRHOIDS AND ANAL FISSURES

Hemorrhoids consist of spongy tissues in the anus that have many blood vessels. If the vessels become enlarged or irritated, they may bleed painlessly. While hemorrhoids are not harmful, one must be sure that the bleeding is not from a cancer.

Anal fissures are small cracks in the lining of the anus. Unlike hemorrhoids, they are usually painful. They may bleed, but the accompanying anal pain distinguishes them from more serious conditions.

COLORECTAL CANCER 3

CHAPTER 4
WHAT CAUSES COLORECTAL CANCER AND HOW CAN IT BE PREVENTED?

RISK FACTORS

It is not yet clear why colorectal cancer develops, but a number of *risk factors* may play a role. Having a risk factor does not mean that you will develop the disease; it just means that you are more likely to develop the disease than someone who does not have the risk factor. Eliminating a risk factor may reduce your chance of developing colorectal cancer. However, it is important to realize that 75% of colorectal cancers develop in individuals with no known risk factors, other than being over the age of 50.

AGE

Increasing age is the single greatest risk factor for colorectal cancer. In essence, the older a person gets, the higher their risk of developing colorectal cancer. It is rare for colorectal cancer to occur in people under the age of 40 unless they have a colorectal cancer hereditary syndrome. In the average population, the risk begins to rise at 40 years of age and then starts to climb precipitously at age 50, doubling with each decade to reach a peak at 70 years. Over 90% of cases of colorectal cancer occur in people over the age of 50. The average age of newly diagnosed colorectal cancer patients is 64.

POLYPS

Polyps are small growths that can develop on the lining of the colon and rectum. Almost all colorectal cancers develop from a type of polyp called an *adenoma*. With time, the cells of some adenomas gradually transform into cancer cells. Adenomas become more common with increasing age. About 5% to 10% of individuals over the age of 50 have one or more. The larger an adenoma gets, the more likely it is to develop into a colorectal cancer. There is about a 1% chance each year that an adenoma polyp will develop into cancer. The longer one lives with an adenoma, the higher the chance that it will become cancerous. It is estimated that a period of five to 15 years is required for the transformation from benign adenoma to colorectal cancer. The removal of adenoma polyps while they are still benign is one of the greatest cancer prevention procedures presently known. A patient who has had polyps removed can form other polyps in later years, so re-examination every few years is required.

OBESITY, SEDENTARY LIFESTYLE, AND DIET

Being overweight increases one's risk of several types of cancer, including colorectal cancer. Excess weight is generally associated with reduced levels of physical activity, increased dietary fat, and overall increased calorie intake. Since these elements are difficult to separate in studies, the individual contribution of each to colorectal cancer risk is hard to determine. For example, diets high in fat are also high in calories and are more likely to be consumed by people who are overweight.

Diets low in fiber and high in red meat have also been linked with colorectal cancer. A substance called *nitrosamide* is found in the feces of people who eat red meat and has been implicated as one possible factor. The role of dietary fiber remains controversial. Colorectal cancer has been associated with diets low in fiber, but recent studies have shown that increasing the amount of fiber may not significantly reduce the risk of colorectal cancer.

PREVIOUS CANCER

People who have already had one colorectal cancer are at a higher than normal risk for developing another one.

FAMILY HISTORY OF CANCER

The chance of developing colorectal cancer increases with the number of immediate relatives (parents, brothers, sisters, or offspring) who have had the disease. Twenty-five percent of those who develop colorectal cancer have a relative that has had it. Ten percent have at least one immediate relative with the disease. However, 75% of those who develop colorectal cancer are the first ones in their family.

RARE HEREDITARY SYNDROMES

There are two main hereditary syndromes for the development of colorectal cancer. The first is called *familial adenomatous polyposis* (FAP). FAP leads to the development of hundreds or thousands of colon polyps. People with FAP must be diagnosed at a very young age if they are to avoid colorectal cancer. The undiagnosed patient with FAP will typically develop colorectal cancer in his or her twenties. It is almost never newly diagnosed in patients over 40 since untreated FAP patients rarely live that long.

The second most notable colorectal cancer hereditary syndrome is called *hereditary non-polyposis colorectal cancer* (HNPCC), also referred to as *Lynch syndrome* or *cancer family syndrome*. HNPCC is different from FAP in that patients develop far fewer polyps. It is a much more common problem, accounting for 3% to 5% of all colorectal cancer. The average age of a patient with HNPCC is 44 years, compared with 64 years in non-hereditary colorectal cancer. HNPCC is also associated with the development of other cancers. The most common associated cancer is cancer of the lining of the uterus (endometrium).

INFLAMMATORY BOWEL DISEASE

The two common forms of inflammatory bowel disease (IBD) are ulcerative colitis and Crohn's disease. People who have had either of these diseases for 8 years or longer are at increased risk of developing colorectal cancer. IBD affects 2% to 6% of North Americans, and in some patients with these diseases, the risk of developing colorectal cancer is five to 10 times greater than similar-aged members of the general population. As the risk of colorectal cancer in IBD varies with type, location, and extent of inflammatory disease, patients with IBD should be guided by specialists in determining their individual risk and the most appropriate way of managing that risk.

OCCUPATIONAL HAZARDS

Environmental and occupational pollutants such as machinist cutting oil, woodworkers' glue, carpet makers' dust, and crop-protective agents have all been linked to colorectal cancer, but the evidence confirming a true cause-and-effect relationship is not strong. The link between asbestos exposure and colorectal cancer is stronger. Studies show a two-fold increase in colorectal cancer for asbestos workers compared to individuals not exposed to asbestos.

CIGARETTE SMOKING, ALCOHOL, PHYSICAL ACTIVITY LEVELS

There is no clear-cut relationship between colon cancer and smoking or alcohol consumption, although there is a fair bit of data that tend to group these lifestyle choices with colorectal cancer. The reason it is difficult to know whether smoking or alcohol are important is because they tend to occur more often in individuals who are sedentary, who tend to have higher fat content in their diet, and who eat less fiber—all potential risk factors for colorectal cancer.

STOOL COMPOSITION

Most compounds that produce colon cancer in animal experiments do not do so in germ-free animals (animals with no bacteria in their feces). This suggests that intestinal bacteria play a role in the cause of colon cancer. What we eat determines the type of feces we produce and the types of bacteria they contain. This may explain the geographical differences in cancer rates since types of bacteria in the colon vary geographically. Some bacteria may be cancer-promoting and others cancer-preventing. Meat eaters have a different pattern of bacterial species than vegetarians.

CAN COLON CANCER BE PREVENTED?

Even though we do not know the exact cause of most colorectal cancers, it is possible to prevent many of them. Here are the ways:

IDENTIFYING AND REMOVING POLYPS

Seventy-five percent of colorectal cancers develop from a particular type of polyp called an *adenoma* (see Chapter 6). Removing adenomas while they are still benign is the most effective way of preventing colorectal cancer. For most people, that means starting a colorectal cancer screening program to look for adenomas, by the age of 50. A screening program uses tests to look for polyps or cancer in patients who have no symptoms. If there is a family history of colorectal cancer or polyps, a screening program may have to be started at a younger age. Check with your doctor.

MANAGING RISK FACTORS

Managing the risk factors that can be controlled, such as diet and exercise, may reduce the chances of developing colorectal cancer. There is now reasonable evidence that increasing physical activity, eating plenty of fruits, vegetables, and whole-grain foods, while limiting intake of high-fat foods and red meat, can reduce cancer risk in general. At least 30 minutes of physical activity on five or more days of the week is recommended. If you are overweight, lose weight until you are at a healthy level and maintain it. Your doctor can help you determine your healthiest weight. Although we can't do anything about advancing age, beginning a screening program to look for polyps or cancer at age 50 can significantly improve our chances of avoiding colorectal cancer.

DIET AND SUPPLEMENTS

Substances in the diet may protect us from cancer. Brussels sprouts, cabbage, turnips, broccoli, and cauliflower have been shown to increase the activity of certain enzymes that protect animals from laboratory-induced colon tumors. Fruits and vegetables, long thought to have a possible protective effect, contain flavinoids, compounds that may be involved in killing old and abnormal cells and inhibiting those cells that can become cancerous.

There is some evidence to suggest that other nutrients may also be beneficial, including foods containing higher amounts of calcium and vitamins A, C, D, and E. In animal experiments, vitamin C and vitamin E appear to have some antitumor effects. However, it is difficult to prove any value in humans. A well-conducted study of antioxidants beta carotene, vitamin C, and vitamin E has shown no effect on colorectal cancer risk. Calcium decreases the likelihood of adenoma polyps, but it has not been proven conclusively that calcium reduces the risk of colorectal cancer or death from the disease.

In a recent study on breast cancer it was accidentally found that women in the study who consumed high levels of the B vitamin folic acid appeared to have a lower risk of colorectal cancer. Folic acid is required for DNA synthesis and it is thought that too little folic acid in the body might lead to mutations and cancer. Folic acid is found in foods such as leafy green vegetables, beans and peas, orange juice, and liver. You can buy the synthetic form of folic acid at most pharmacies.

High levels of selenium in the soil and foliage have been correlated with lower rates of colon cancer in certain geographic areas of the United States.

Selenium fed to animals protects against laboratory-induced cancer. Broccoli contains high levels of selenium.

Several carefully conducted studies have shown that acetylsalicylic acid (ASA or Aspirin) or certain anti-inflammatory drugs called NSAIDs (sulindac and celecoxib) slow the development of adenoma polyps in people with FAP, a hereditary disease characterized by many colon polyps and early colorectal cancer (see Chapter 42). However, no good trial has shown that NSAIDs prevent deaths from colorectal cancer, and at least one well-reputed trial showed no association between ASA use and the incidence of colorectal cancer. Furthermore, it has recently been found that certain types of NSAIDs, particularly those in the COX-2 inhibitor family such as celecoxib (Celebrex), are harmful to the cardiovascular system and cannot now be recommended for use in any polyp or colorectal cancer prevention program.

In summary, there are numerous claims for and against many foods and supplements when it comes to preventing colorectal cancer. It would be comforting to know that such simple measures could protect us. But most claims in these areas cannot be or have not yet been substantiated by critical academic research. At the present time, two things are certain. No food or supplement has been shown to reduce death from colorectal cancer, and none has been shown to be as effective in reducing death from colorectal cancer as a colorectal cancer screening program that uses tests to look for polyps or cancer in patients who do not have symptoms.

UNDERSTANDING AND MANAGING HEREDITARY FACTORS

Family history cannot be controlled, but understanding the implications of having a family history of colorectal cancer is the first step in developing an effective strategy against the disease. Particular patterns of colorectal cancer occurring in a family suggest an underlying hereditary predisposition. A combination of careful testing (screening) and genetic testing, when warranted, can help prevent colorectal cancer in almost every case.

CHAPTER 5
HOW COMMON IS COLORECTAL CANCER AND WHAT IS MY RISK?

Colorectal cancer is the second leading cause of death from cancer in North America. Only lung cancer causes more cancer deaths. Among non-smokers, colorectal cancer is number one.

One-quarter of all North Americans are at risk because of increased age and other risk factors. In 2005, over 60,000 people in North America will die from colorectal cancer, leaving behind more than 600,000 potential years of life lost (based on an average of 10 years lost per person). Approximately 150,000 new cases will be diagnosed. More women over the age of 75 will die from colorectal cancer than from breast cancer.

In Canada, an estimated 19,000 people will develop colorectal cancer in 2005 and 8,300 will die of it. At these rates, one in 15 Canadians will get the disease at some point in their lifetime and one in 28 will die of it.

GOOD NEWS AND BAD NEWS

The good news is that there are fewer colorectal cancers appearing per

100,000 people (a lower incidence) and the cure rates are improving. This would seem to imply that colorectal cancer should be becoming less of a problem. However, the bad news is that, because of the growth and aging of the population, the total number of new cases has continued to rise steadily and significantly among both men and women. For reasons unknown, the improvement in cure rates has occurred more in women than in men.

WHAT PARTS OF THE COLON ARE MOST AFFECTED?

Colorectal cancer occurs most often in the first half of the colon (cecum, ascending colon, and transverse colon), followed by the rectum, and it occurs least often in the descending and sigmoid colon. As age increases, the numbers of patients with cancer in the rectum declines, leading to a higher percentage of patients with cancer in the first half of the colon. These changes have implications with regard to tests designed to look for colorectal cancer since, as age increases, the importance of examining the first half of the colon becomes more important.

THE EFFECT OF PLACE OF RESIDENCE

Incidence (the number of colorectal cancers per 100,000 people) and rates of death (mortality rates) from colorectal cancer vary with place of residence. The variation across the provinces is shown in Tables 1 and 2. In Canada, incidence rates are slightly higher in the eastern provinces than the western provinces, for both men and women. An east-west difference is not as notable in mortality rates, although BC and Alberta do have the lowest mortality rates in Canada. Several factors must be considered when interpreting inter-provincial differences. For example, certain risk factors may be more prevalent in some provinces than in others. Types of foods consumed, age of population, the availability of screening programs, and so on are not consistent across the country.

TABLE 1. ESTIMATED AGE-STANDARDIZED INCIDENCE RATES FOR COLORECTAL CANCER BY PROVINCE, CANADA 2004 (PER 100,000 POPULATION).

	CAN	NF	PE	NS	NB	QC	ON	MB	SK	AB	BC
Male	62	80	64	72	64	66	61	65	57	56	56
Female	41	47	52	50	47	41	42	43	37	37	36

SOURCE: NATIONAL CANCER INSTITUTE OF CANADA

TABLE 2. ESTIMATED AGE-STANDARDIZED MORTALITY RATES (DEATH RATES) FROM COLORECTAL CANCER BY PROVINCE, CANADA 2004 (PER 100,000 POPULATION).

	CAN	NF	PE	NS	NB	QC	ON	MB	SK	AB	BC
Male	27	36	32	30	27	32	26	30	26	23	22
Female	17	26	23	24	17	14	17	18	15	13	14

SOURCE: NATIONAL CANCER INSTITUTE OF CANADA

WHAT IS MY RISK?

In assessing one's own risk, the two key elements most important to consider are age and family history.

THE AGE FACTOR

Except in those with hereditary colorectal cancer (see Chapter 42), colorectal cancer is a disease of older people. For men and women in their 70s, the probability of developing colorectal cancer in the next 10 years is 2% to 3%, which is about 10 times greater than for those in their 40s (0.2%). Table 3 lists the probability of developing colorectal cancer within the next 10 years, by age. Table 4 lists the lifetime probability of developing and dying from colorectal cancer.

TABLE 3. PROBABILITY (%) OF DEVELOPING COLORECTAL CANCER WITHIN THE NEXT 10 YEARS, BY AGE.

	30-39 YRS	40-49 YRS	50-59 YRS	60-69 YRS	70-79 YRS	80-89YRS
Male	0.1	0.2	0.8	2.1	3.4	3.3
Female	–	0.2	0.6	1.3	2.3	3.0

SOURCE: NATIONAL CANCER INSTITUTE OF CANADA, 2004

TABLE 4. LIFETIME PROBABILITY OF DEVELOPING AND DYING FROM COLORECTAL CANCER.

	DEVELOPING COLORECTAL CANCER	DYING FROM COLORECTAL CANCER
Male	7.2% (1 in 14)	3.6% (1 in 28)
Female	6.5% (1 in 15)	3.2% (1 in 31)

SOURCE: NATIONAL CANCER INSTITUTE OF CANADA, 2004

THE FAMILY HISTORY FACTOR

Numerous studies confirm that immediate (first-degree) relatives (daughter, son, sister, brother, parent) of colorectal cancer patients are themselves at a two- to threefold increased risk of colorectal cancer. The majority of these cases are not part of any clear-cut hereditary syndrome.

Having a family history of colorectal cancer also appears to influence the age of onset of colorectal cancer. People who have a first-degree relative with colorectal cancer tend to develop the disease (if they are going to get it) about 10 years earlier than other people with colorectal cancer. This increased cancer risk caused by a family history of colorectal cancer disappears by age 60, so that if one has not developed the cancer by then, the risk is similar to the general public at the same age.

TABLE 5. ESTIMATED LIFETIME RISK OF DEVELOPING COLORECTAL CANCER BASED UPON FAMILY HISTORY.

FAMILY HISTORY	LIFETIME RISK OF COLORECTAL CANCER
No family history of colorectal cancer	2%
One first-degree relative (parent, sibling, child)	6%
One first-degree and two second-degree relatives	8%
One first-degree relative under 45 years	10%
Two first-degree relatives	17%
HNPCC mutation carrier (hereditary syndrome—see Chapter 42)	70%
FAP mutation carrier (hereditary syndrome—see Chapter 42)	100%

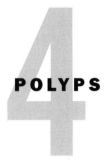

POLYPS

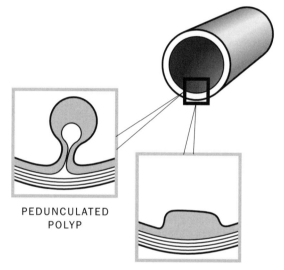

COLON SECTION

PEDUNCULATED
POLYP

SESSILE POLYP

Figure 9. *Polyp shape.*

CHAPTER 6
WHAT ARE POLYPS AND
HOW ARE THEY TREATED?

A *polyp* is simply a lump projecting above the surface of the intestinal lining, the *mucosa*. Polyps come in a variety of types; some are important and some are not. They also come in different shapes and sizes. Polyps that have a stalk and head are called *pedunculated* shaped polyps (Figure 9). Polyps that are flat, without a stalk, are called *sessile* shaped polyps. Doctors pay close attention to polyps because it is believed that 95% or more of colorectal cancers originate in polyps. However, not all polyps have the potential to become malignant.

HARMLESS POLYPS

HYPERPLASTIC POLYPS

Hyperplastic polyps are the most common form of intestinal polyp and are not related to cancer. They are small, less than five mm (¼ inch) in diameter, pale gray, flat bumps found on the lining of the large bowel and particularly in the rectum. They are caused by a build-up of intestinal lining cells. These cells will often just slough off, so an examiner may see a hyperplastic polyp one week and not the next. Reliable naked eye distinction of hyperplastic polyps from more significant polyps is not always possible, so they should be removed or a sample of the tissue removed for an accurate diagnosis. It is currently believed that hyperplastic polyps have no potential to become cancers, so they require neither treatment nor follow-up if the diagnosis is certain.

INFLAMMATORY POLYPS

Inflammatory polyps are the result of inflammation in the colon or rectum from infection or inflammatory diseases of the bowel. Inflammatory polyps have no potential to become malignant (although there is an increased risk of colon cancer among people with long-standing ulcerative colitis). Inflammatory polyps may go away on their own if the colon inflammation improves.

HAMARTOMATOUS POLYPS

Hamartomatous polyps consist of normal cells arranged in an abnormal, disorganized fashion. The abnormality is present at birth but the polyps themselves may not become apparent until the tissue grows large enough for a lump to form. Most authorities believe that hamartomatous polyps do not become cancerous.

JUVENILE POLYPS

Juvenile polyps, also called *retention polyps*, are seen predominantly in children aged one to seven. These harmless polyps consist of a collection of mucus glands. They can bleed or slough. In rare cases there may be multiple polyps (*juvenile polyposis*) that may be associated with cancer.

LYMPHOID POLYPS

Lymphoid polyps consist of harmless collections of lymphoid cells, one of the types of white blood cells. Occasionally they can be seen in association with other lymphatic disease, so careful assessment by a pathologist is important.

POTENTIALLY HARMFUL POLYPS—THE ADENOMAS

Adenomas (adenomatous polyps) are the polyps that have the potential to become cancers, so it is with these that we are primarily concerned (Figure a, color section). Adenomas become more common with increasing age. About 5% to 10% of individuals over the age of 50 have one or more adenomas. The larger an adenoma gets, the more likely it is to develop into a colorectal cancer. There is about a 1% chance each year that an adenoma polyp will develop into cancer in an individual, and the longer one lives with an adenomatous polyp, the higher the chance that it will become cancerous. It is estimated that five to 15 years is required for the transformation from benign adenoma to colorectal cancer.

REMOVING POLYPS

REMOVING A POLYP THROUGH A SCOPE—POLYPECTOMY

Most polyps are removed through a scope, generally a *colonoscope* (Figure 10, Figures b and c, color section). The procedure is called *colonoscopic polypectomy*. The special tool used to perform a polypectomy through a scope is called a *polypectomy snare*. The polypectomy snare consists of a plastic sheath that contains a wire loop (Figure d series, color section). The snare is passed down the operating channel of the colonoscope and the wire loop is maneuvered over the polyp. The operator then gently withdraws the wire loop back into the plastic sheath to tighten the wire loop around the stalk of the polyp. As the loop is tightening, an electrical current is sent down the wire, cauterizing (that is, searing shut) the stalk as the wire cuts through it (Figure e series, color section). The amputated polyp can then be grasped and removed. Multiple polyps can be removed during one procedure.

Colonoscopic polypectomy is not risk-free, but the alternative of formal surgery to remove the polyp usually involves even greater risk. Unless the polyp is too large or flat, or is thought to already be a small cancer, colonoscopic

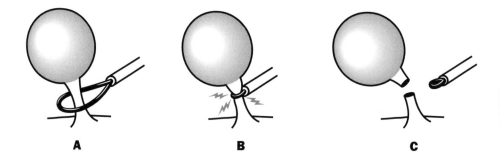

Figure 10. *A polyp removed by a colonoscopy snare.*

polypectomy is usually attempted. The examiner must judge whether it is safe to go ahead with a colonoscopic polypectomy. The risks of polypectomy are bleeding and perforation (making a hole in the colon). The probability of perforation or bleeding is one in 500 cases (by comparison, the risk of perforation in simple colonoscopy without polypectomy is one in 3,000). If the bowel is perforated, surgery to repair the hole is usually required. If bleeding is encountered when removing a polyp, it can usually be managed by cauterizing the bleeding vessel through the colonoscope or simply by having the patient rest and allowing the bleeding to stop on its own while the patient is carefully supervised.

REMOVING A POLYP AT SURGERY

Polyps sometimes need to be removed in the operating room if they are too large or flat to be removed through a scope, or if they appear to have already turned into cancer.

THE VERY LARGE POLYP

Colonoscopists will consider removing a very large polyp in pieces, provided that it looks benign. The snare is used to repeatedly carve off portions of the polyp until it is completely gone. The risk of bleeding during this type of removal is greater than during a simple polypectomy around a stalk.

THE VERY FLAT POLYP

Very flat polyps pose an increased risk for perforation if attempts are made to remove them with a colonoscopy snare. The snare, when tightened, has no stalk to grasp and may, instead, grasp the underlying bowel wall and cut through it. If this makes a hole in the bowel, a surgical repair is required. Sometimes a flat polyp can be more easily removed if the colonoscopist first injects salt water (saline) underneath its surface to cause it to rise up off the underlying bowel wall, permitting the snare to get a better hold around the polyp while leaving the deeper bowel wall unaffected.

THE VILLOUS ADENOMA OF THE RECTUM

A *villous adenoma* is a special kind of flat, broad-based polyp. These polyps are so broad that they can literally encircle the entire lining of a portion of the bowel, carpeting it with polyp tissue. The most common location for the villous adenoma is in the rectum. If they are not removed in one piece with a margin of normal tissue around them, they often come back. The best way to remove them is in the operating room, directly through the anus (Figure 11). The older method of cauterizing or trying to burn off a villous adenoma leads to almost certain recurrence and should no longer be done. Villous adenomas of the rectum have a tendency to recur so it is important that the rectum be carefully examined by the surgeon every six months for up to five years after surgery. Then, re-excision can be done promptly if any villous adenoma tissue reappears.

THE POLYP THAT CONTAINS CANCER

Sometimes a pathologist will find cancer in a polyp removed by colonoscopic polypectomy. Such a polyp is called a *malignant polyp*. Managing the malignant polyp is discussed in Chapter 24 in the section of Special Surgical Considerations.

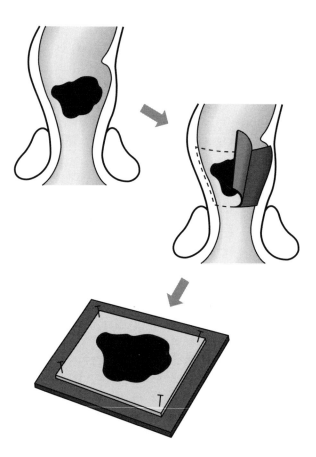

Figure 11. *Removing a villous adenoma of the rectum. The villous adenoma is carefully removed through the anus and pinned out on a cork board to retain its shape. The pathologist will look for a good margin of normal lining around the polyp to ensure that no abnormal tissue remains.*

FOLLOW-UP AFTER REMOVING A POLYP

No follow-up is required if a removed polyp is diagnosed as a hyperplastic polyp. If, however, the polyp is an adenoma, it means that the patient is at increased risk for additional adenomas in the future and colorectal cancer as a result. Therefore, people who have an adenoma removed need follow-up colonoscopy at regular intervals for as long as they remain healthy. A follow-up colonoscopy should be performed three years later and every three years thereafter if additional polyps are found. If no further polyps are identified at any colonoscopy, the follow-up colonoscopy testing can be extended to every five years. If the removed polyp shows evidence of cancer, or is incompletely removed, an initial recheck of the polypectomy site should be undertaken six months to one year following the initial polypectomy and then repeated at a frequency determined by the specialist.

5

EARLY DETECTION OF COLORECTAL CANCER

CHAPTER 7
SCREENING TESTS FOR
COLORECTAL CANCER

WHAT IS SCREENING?

By the time symptoms appear, cancer may be well-established and, in many cases, may have already spread to other parts of the body. In order to maximize the chances of cure, colorectal cancer must be identified in its earliest phases, before symptoms occur. *Screening* is the process of looking for a disease (in this case, colorectal cancer) in individuals who have no symptoms. Screening is particularly useful in colorectal cancer since polyps, the initial form of this disease, usually exist undetected for many years before they cause trouble.

Screening reduces deaths from colorectal cancer. The consensus among authorities is that screening for colorectal cancer should begin routinely at the age of 50 in those of average risk, and younger when there is a strong family history.

THE SCREENING TESTS

There are a variety of tests that can be used to detect the presence of colorectal cancer or its early form, polyps. The different tests range from being somewhat insensitive (meaning the test will miss a percentage of people who do have polyps or colorectal cancer) to those that are highly accurate. The more insensitive tests are convenient, harmless, and inexpensive while the highly accurate ones cost more and involve some risk.

FECAL OCCULT BLOOD TEST

Polyps and cancers may bleed in amounts too small to be seen by the naked eye. This invisible bleeding is known as *occult bleeding. Fecal occult blood tests* are designed to identify minute quantities of blood or blood breakdown products in the stool that are too small to be seen. Fecal occult blood testing is the most widely used screening test for colorectal cancer. It fulfills the requirements of a screening test for large populations in that it is inexpensive, easy, not embarrassing, painless, and convenient. It is not particularly sensitive, so some people with significant polyps or colorectal cancer will be missed by this test. Nor is it very specific, which means that some people will show a false positive test and need to undergo further tests before ultimately being proven normal. Still, several reliable studies have shown that, when used on large numbers of people, yearly fecal occult blood testing reduces colorectal cancer deaths by as much as 33%.

There are a number of fecal occult blood tests available. Most require the patient to take a small sample of fresh stool and smear it onto one of three different panels of a card with testing chemicals in it (Figure f, color section). In the laboratory, a few drops of hydrogen peroxide are added to each panel and the card is then examined for a color change that signals the presence of minute quantities of blood. Because bleeding may be intermittent, the most common way of doing the test is to use one panel for each consecutive bowel movement. A test result is considered positive if any of the three panels test positive.

Fecal occult blood tests may be affected by a variety of substances in the diet. A blood enzyme (peroxidase) that the test is designed to detect may be mimicked by the contents of certain foods such as turnips, horse-radish, broccoli, cauliflower, and radishes. Meat products may also give false-positive results. Vitamin C may interfere by blocking the chemical reaction, leading to a false-negative result (a negative test even when there is blood in the stool). For reliable results, patients must follow a special diet designed to minimize false-positive and false-negative results.

Typically, 1% to 5% of a general population will test positive with fecal occult blood tests, but up to 85% of patients with a positive test will ultimately be proven, through further testing, to have nothing wrong. Another weakness of the test is that it will be positive in only 37% to 69% of patients with an abnormality. Some patients, therefore, will have a false-negative test, meaning that the test was negative but they actually have disease. A false-negative test can provide false security to individuals who really do have cancer, contributing to a delay in further testing and accurate diagnosis.

DIGITAL RECTAL EXAM

A digital rectal exam (DRE) is a simple procedure performed in the doctor's office as part of a routine physical examination. The physician inserts a lubricated, gloved finger through the anus and up into the lower rectum to feel for abnormalities. A cancer of the rectum has the consistency of firm rubber, quite different from the surrounding normal tissues.

While simple to do, the digital rectal exam is the least sensitive screening method because it is restricted physically to such a short distance (a negative result does not exclude the possibility of rectal cancer). Also, the usefulness of this type of screening is limited by the experience of the physician.

SCOPE (ENDOSCOPE) TESTS

A variety of instruments are available for looking into the bowel. Collectively, these instruments are called *endoscopes* (endo meaning inside). The instruments may be rigid or flexible, varying in length from 25 cm (10 inches) to 160 cm (63 inches).

Rigid sigmoidoscopy

The most common type of endoscope, the rigid sigmoidoscope, is a 25 cm (10 inch) long rigid metal or plastic viewing tube that the examiner passes through the anus in order to examine the rectum (Figure 12, Figure g color section). The procedure is called *rigid sigmoidoscopy* or *proctoscopy* or *proctosigmoidoscopy*. While approximately 30% of polyps and cancers develop within the 25 cm region of the bowel theoretically reached by the rigid sigmoidoscope, it is rarely practical to go the full 25 cm due to patient discomfort. An examined distance of 10 to 13 cm (four to five inches) likely represents what most clinicians accomplish with this instrument. Therefore the value of rigid sigmoidoscopy is probably over-estimated.

However, the rigid sigmoidoscope has been shown to significantly reduce death from colorectal cancer within the part that it does examine. Rigid sigmoidoscopy is generally carried out in the doctor's office, without sedation. Some physicians prepare the patient ahead of time with one or two enemas. Others do this test without any bowel preparation. It is an unpleasant and embarrassing experience for most patients, but it should not be painful. The examination should not proceed beyond the patient's level of comfort, and so rarely is the entire instrument inserted. If a higher examination is necessary, a different test is required.

Flexible sigmoidoscopy

Flexible sigmoidoscopy involves the use of a flexible 60 cm (24 inch) instrument that can bend around the corners of the bowel and go higher than the rigid instrument (Figure h color section). Approximately 55% of polyps and cancers develop within the reach of a 60 cm flexible sigmoidoscope. An expert examiner can assess more than 60 cm of bowel with this instrument since its

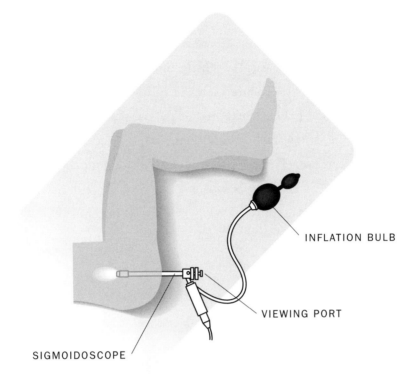

Figure 12. *A patient lying on his side undergoing a rigid sigmoidoscopy examination.*

flexibility can be used to draw down the bowel and accordion it over the scope. Flexible sigmoidoscopy requires some bowel preparation, usually consisting of two enemas shortly before the procedure. Sometimes, an oral bowel washout is prescribed by the physician. Sedation is rarely used. The test is reasonably safe; the rate of perforation of the bowel by the scope is one in 6,000. In a number of studies, flexible sigmoidoscopy has been shown to reduce the colorectal cancer death rate by up to 85% within the range of examination.

Flexible sigmoidoscopy is, in theory, a simple office procedure that can be done without any patient sedation, and it is frequently recommended as a screening method (combined with fecal occult blood testing). However, for a number of reasons, it does not seem to work out in many cases. First, a flexible sigmoidoscope is a very expensive device, and most physicians cannot afford to buy and maintain one for their office. Second, disinfecting the instrument between patients is costly, time-consuming, and requires special expertise. The procedure itself can be quite painful and considerable experience and finesse is required of the physician. Most examiners are unable to insert the full 60 cm of the scope. Last, it still leaves over half (and in most cases much more than half) of the colon unseen. Many clinicians feel that, given all these drawbacks, they would prefer having an expert do a full colonoscopy (see below) to review the entire colon and rectum. For these reasons, flexible sigmoidoscopy is not readily available in many parts of the country.

Colonoscopy

A colonoscope is a 160 cm (63 inch) flexible scope. It is long enough to permit examination of the entire rectum and colon in most cases (Figure b, color section). Bowel preparation by oral agents is required (see Appendix), and intravenous sedation is given to keep the patient comfortable during the procedure.

Studies show that colonoscopy reduces the number of deaths from colorectal cancer, but the studies are of lower quality than those studies confirming the value of fecal occult blood testing. In practice, the proportion of cancers that develop in the region viewed by a colonoscope is an estimated 95%, since it is not always possible to get the colonoscope all the way through the colon and even an experienced colonoscopist can sometimes miss a problem. The false-positive rate for colonoscopy is negligible because the examiner is looking directly at the bowel wall, can easily distinguish normal from abnormal, and is unlikely to mistake a piece of feces for a polyp. Biopsies (samples) of suspicious lesions can be taken directly through the scope. In addition, polyps can usually be removed through the colonoscope.

Colonoscopy is a low risk procedure, but it is not zero risk. The risk of perforation of the bowel by the colonoscope is one in 3,000. Risk of damage or bleeding during removal of a polyp is one in 500. There is no radiation with colonoscopy, although some physicians occasionally take simple X-rays to determine the position of the scope if they are having difficulty.

The procedure takes anywhere from 10 to 40 minutes, depending upon how easily the bowel accepts the instrument, the skill of the examiner, and what needs to be done during the examination. It is carried out in a specially equipped *endoscopy suite* in a hospital or clinic. Most colonoscopes now produce a video image that is shown on a television monitor in the procedure room. The doctor (and sometimes the patient) watches the monitor to see the image of the inside of the colon.

As the instrument makes its way into the bowel, the doctor looks for abnormalities such as polyps, cancers, or areas of inflammation. Grasping instruments may be passed down a channel in the colonoscope to allow the physician to remove a tissue sample of suspicious areas.

When the procedure is over, the instrument is removed and the patient is asked to remain lying down until the effects of the sedation have worn off sufficiently. The average patient is ready to go home about 90 minutes after the sedative injection. However, subtle effects of the medication can last for a number of hours longer, so the patient should not drive home or engage in any other potentially dangerous activity until the next day. Arrangements should be made ahead of time for the patient to be taken home by a friend or relative.

If polyps are removed during the colonoscopy, some doctors will instruct the patient to remain on a clear fluid diet for the rest of the day. Otherwise, a normal diet may be resumed after the patient has recovered from sedation.

DIAGNOSTIC IMAGING STUDIES

(NON-SCOPE TESTS USED TO VISUALIZE THE BODY)

Barium enema

A *barium enema* is a special X-ray of the colon. Complete bowel preparation (see Appendix) is required prior to a barium enema since it is difficult to distinguish stool from polyps in an X-ray.

During a barium enema, the patient lies on a flat X-ray table, and a small rubber tube is placed into the anus. Barium is pumped gently through the tube into the rectum and colon. No sedation is used. Barium appears white on the X-ray film while the other tissue of the abdomen appears black (Figure i, color section). The patient may be asked to turn over onto one or the other side and some gentle pressure may be applied to the abdomen to better define a specific part of the colon. Anywhere from five to 15 X-rays are taken to show the colon and rectum at various angles. The insertion of some air with the barium (air-contrast barium enema) can enhance the view.

A barium enema can reveal about 85% to 92% of large bowel lesions. It is less accurate than colonoscopy and there are no studies proving that barium enemas reduce deaths from colorectal cancer. Unlike examinations that involve direct viewing of the bowel (sigmoidoscopy and colonoscopy), it is difficult to tell the difference between a bit of stool and a polyp during a barium enema because the radiologist is only seeing the shape of something in the colon. In about 10% of barium enema examinations, the radiologist will recommend further tests (usually colonoscopy) to clarify a potential abnormality.

A barium enema does involve radiation but barium itself does not emit X-rays, neither is it radioactive. The amount of radiation is about twice what we get normally during the course of a year. After the X-ray, residual barium normally passes out of the rectum without difficulty. If the barium is not expelled, it can harden in the colon, leading to constipation. The radiologist may prescribe a simple enema to help patients expel the barium after the procedure, particularly if the patient is prone to constipation.

Virtual colonoscopy (colonography)

Computerized tomographic (CT) *colonography* or *virtual colonoscopy* is a relatively new technique used to examine the colon (Figure j, color section). The technique involves an oral bowel preparation, as in colonoscopy. After this, a small tube is placed into the patient's rectum, and carbon dioxide is introduced into the colon to distend it. The patient's colon is then viewed with a specially equipped CT scanner.

One of the main advantages of virtual colonoscopy is that it is minimally invasive; no long scope is passed into the colon, and no intravenous or other sedation is required. The procedure is also fast, and patients can usually resume normal activities immediately after the appointment. Moreover, the CT images include structures outside the bowel wall, so the radiologist might find other disease that has nothing to do with the colon.

The disadvantages are that a full bowel preparation is still required, and that no biopsy is possible. If an abnormality is discovered with virtual colonoscopy, the patient is referred for colonoscopy. In addition, the test does require some radiation, about twice the radiation of a barium enema.

The sensitivity of virtual colonoscopy for identifying polyps is not well known at this time. There have been two large studies on virtual colonoscopy published. The first suggested that it was very good and the second suggested that it was not. Critics of the first study say that the radiologists were highly trained and motivated and likely did not reflect the results that general radiologists would ultimately obtain. Critics of the second study claim that the radiologists were inexperienced and the equipment used was not adequate.

As in all new investigations, it will take some years before the true value of virtual colonoscopy is known. For the present time it is important that patients who wish to have a virtual colonoscopy ensure that the facility has a multi-detector CT scanner (at least four detectors), and an established virtual colonoscopy program with experienced virtual colonoscopy radiologists. Ideally, the facility should also have an arrangement with a colonoscopy facility to allow immediate referral when biopsy or polyp removal is necessary, thus avoiding an additional bowel preparation.

FECAL DNA ANALYSIS

This test is based on the fact that colorectal cancers probably shed cancer cells into the stool. Fecal DNA analysis identifies abnormal DNA (genetic material) from the shed colorectal cancer cells. When this test is positive, there is almost certainly a cancer in the bowel. Unfortunately, it misses a large percentage of patients with colorectal cancer. The first big trial of a fecal DNA analysis showed that while it did find more cancers than fecal occult blood testing, it found just half of the colon and rectal cancers detected by colonoscopy. The test is expensive and is not currently available in most centers.

WHICH TEST BEST SUITS MY NEEDS?

The wide array of screening tests can be confusing to patients at first. With the guidance of your physician and the information in the following chapter, you should be able to confidently make an informed decision.

CHAPTER 8
WHICH SCREENING TEST IS BEST?

When considering the use of either fecal occult blood screening, flexible sigmoidoscopy, colonoscopy, barium enema, or virtual colonoscopy, it becomes apparent that each test has advocates who consider it superior. Determining which test is the best depends upon who is doing the judging. For academics, scientific proof that a test saves lives may be the only real consideration. For those organizing screening programs for large populations, safety and low cost are the key. For individuals seeking personal screening, accuracy, safety, and comfort are most important. Each test finds cancers; some more effectively than others, but with added benefits comes the potential for increased discomfort, harm, and cost.

WHICH TEST HAS BEEN MOST SCIENTIFICALLY PROVEN TO BE OF BENEFIT?

It has now been proven that screening for colorectal cancer with fecal occult blood tests significantly lowers the rate of death from the disease. In fact, such testing may actually prevent cancer by identifying polyps as well.

The methods of statistical analysis used to assess the value of sigmoidoscopy are considerably weaker, although these studies do suggest that sigmoidoscopy lowers death rates from colorectal cancer. No direct evidence proves that whole-bowel screening (colonoscopy or barium enema) reduces death rates from colorectal cancer, and so some experts consider it too soon to endorse a program of whole-bowel screening. Others feel that since there is some evidence that sigmoidoscopy reduces deaths, it naturally follows that complete bowel examination would save even more lives. They claim it is unethical to wait for scientific certainty.

WHICH TEST IS MOST ACCURATE?

Colonoscopy is the gold standard when it comes to accuracy (see Table 6). It enables inspection of the entire colon, detection of almost all important abnormalities, eliminates the possibility of false positives, and is the only test that permits removal of polyps and the taking of tissue samples. Barium enema also provides a view of the whole colon but is less accurate. The major disadvantage of colonoscopy is that one can not get all the way to the cecum in every case. The *completion rate* (that is, the percentage of colonoscopies in which the physician goes all the way around the colon) varies from 75% to 95%. This can have a major impact on the real accuracy of colonoscopy. Thin females are the most difficult to complete.

Flexible sigmoidoscopy is as accurate as colonoscopy within the length that it can examine, but it is not readily available or well done in many clinics owing to its cost and required expertise. Fecal occult blood screening misses a lot of people with colon cancer, often suggests disease when there is none, and must be repeated every year.

Recent research suggests that virtual colonoscopy (colonography) may match colonoscopy's ability to find polyps that are one cm or larger, but it may also show things that are not really there, giving false-positives.

WHICH TEST IS SAFEST?

Fecal occult blood testing is undoubtedly the safest. At the risk of sounding glib, the only real safety issue is that one could potentially fall into the toilet when attempting to retrieve the specimen. The perforation rate for barium enema is very low, about one in 10,000 cases, but when this occurs it may be lethal. Perforation from colonoscopy is less rare, in the order of one in 3,000 cases, but death has rarely been reported when it occurs. Death from any cause occurs in one in 10,000 colonoscopies. Perforation during flexible sigmoidoscopy is reported at one in 6,000 cases.

The problem with screening tests that could possibly hurt people or even be fatal is that there must be proof that the potential benefit of the test outweighs the possible harm the test might cause. Given that the rate of death from colorectal cancer among persons 50 to 54 years of age is only 1.8 per 10,000 people, one can see that the number of persons harmed by screening could offset the number who benefit. This downside explains the reluctance of some experts to recommend colonoscopy as the preferred colorectal cancer screening test.

WHICH TEST IS MOST COST-EFFECTIVE?

Looking after patients who have advanced colorectal cancer is very expensive. Many studies have shown that every colorectal screening test, including colonoscopy, can save money in the long run. Though colonoscopy is the most expensive test, it may ultimately cost less than the others because it prevents more cancers, does not produce false-positive results that need to be followed by other costly tests, and does not need to be performed very often.

WHAT ABOUT PATIENT PREFERENCES?

Factors influencing patients' choice often depend upon issues that are more subtle than bleeding and perforation rates. Patients also consider such things as preparation and recovery time, discomfort, embarrassment, and the unpleasantness associated with bowel preparation. Other issues include access to specialists, out-of-pocket costs, previous experience with a test, and perceived risk of cancer. For example, a patient might reject a colonoscopy at 50, but feel differently at 65 when the risk of colorectal cancer is higher.

CAN WE START WITH A SIMPLER TEST?

Some feel that an initial flexible sigmoidoscopy is a reasonable way of determining whether colonoscopy should be used. People with abnormalities discovered with flexible sigmoidoscopy are more likely to have additional abnormalities higher up, so flexible sigmoidoscopy can serve as a step prior to full colonoscopy in such patients. However, some patients who are normal within the range of a flexible sigmoidoscope will have a polyp or cancer higher in the colon. Up to 50% of patients with advanced higher abnormalities will be missed if an abnormal flexible sigmoidoscopy is required as a prerequisite for a colonoscopy. This may be reduced to 24% if fecal occult blood testing is done before the flexible sigmoidoscopy since those with a positive occult blood test would skip the flexible sigmoidoscopy and have a colonoscopy instead.

TABLE 6. LIKELIHOOD OF IDENTIFYING AN ABNORMALITY WHEN ONE EXISTS.

Colonoscopy	95%–97%
Virtual colonoscopy (colonography)	*
Barium enema	85%–92%
Flexible sigmoidoscopy & fecal occult blood testing	75%
Flexible sigmoidoscopy alone	50%
Fecal occult blood testing only	15%–55%
Rigid sigmoidoscopy	10%–30%

* FURTHER STUDIES NEEDED

WHAT IS THE CURRENT STATUS OF VIRTUAL COLONOSCOPY?

Virtual colonoscopy continues to be evaluated. Its safe, non-invasive nature is a powerful asset. However, the expense is daunting, and in most jurisdictions, virtual colonoscopy is not yet an insured service. Also, even radiologists who perform virtual colonoscopy recognize that traditional colonoscopy is the gold standard in terms of accuracy and the opportunity it gives the physician to remove polyps.

Still, virtual colonoscopy can likely identify more abnormalities than fecal occult blood testing or flexible sigmoidoscopy, and even critics admit that it outperforms the barium enema. For the time being though, it should be considered an alternative screening method helpful for those who wish to have their whole colon viewed but who are unable or refuse to undergo a standard colonoscopy. And it is an option only for those who have the financial means to pay for it.

WHICH TEST IS BEST?

Those who feel that one specific screening test for colorectal cancer is best are basing their opinion on what they consider to be the highest priority for a screening test. As previously stated, the tests differ in scientific validity, accuracy, magnitude of benefit, safety, cost, feasibility, and so on. No single test is perfect. The right test for one person may be the wrong test for somebody else. Ultimately, the choice of which test is best belongs to the patient who, through consultation with the physician, can choose which procedure best suits his or her needs. Given that over 60% of eligible patients have never had any screening test for this very important and preventable cancer, the "best test" as Dr. S.H. Woolf wrote in the *New England Journal of Medicine* in 2000, may simply be the one that they agree to take.

The following guidelines are reasonable for individuals who want to set up a personal colorectal cancer screening program. They are not designed for large populations. Cost is considered, but not as a priority. The advantages and disadvantages of each screening method have been considered, including what is known about their accuracy and safety. It assumes that most people are willing to travel a modest distance to an expert for these studies given that they are infrequent. These guidelines are only a suggestion. No book or information source can take the place of individual guidance from a physician. After reading this chapter, consult with your physician to determine which screening program is best for you.

PEOPLE AT AVERAGE RISK

People at average risk are defined as age 50 or greater, with no intestinal symptoms, a normal physical examination, an absence of family history of colorectal cancer or colorectal polyps, and a negative fecal occult blood test.

RECOMMENDED SCREENING PROGRAM

Colonoscopy every 10 years starting at the age of 50.

SECOND CHOICE

Annual fecal occult blood test plus flexible sigmoidoscopy every five years starting at the age of 50.

PEOPLE AT MODERATELY INCREASED RISK

People at moderately increased risk are defined as those having one first-degree relative (mother, father, or sibling) with colorectal cancer diagnosed at age 60 or older.

RECOMMENDED SCREENING PROGRAM

Colonoscopy every five years starting at age 40.

SECOND CHOICE

No alternative screening strategies are considered adequate.

PEOPLE AT HIGH RISK WITH NO KNOWN HEREDITARY SYNDROME

People at high-risk with no known hereditary syndrome are defined as those with two or more first-degree relatives (mother, father, or sibling) with colorectal cancer diagnosed at age 60 or younger.

RECOMMENDED SCREENING PROGRAM

Colonoscopy is recommended starting at age 40, or 10 years less than the youngest affected relative, whichever is earlier. Colonoscopy should be repeated every three to five years.

SECOND CHOICE

No alternative screening strategies are considered adequate.

PEOPLE WHO ARE MEMBERS OF FAMILIES WITH KNOWN OR SUSPECTED HEREDITARY COLORECTAL CANCER SYNDROMES

Familial adenomatous polyposis (FAP) is characterized by the early development of hundreds or thousands of colorectal polyps and colorectal cancer. Hereditary non-polyposis colorectal cancer (HNPCC) is characterized by the early development of colorectal cancer but without the numbers of polyps seen in FAP. People with such a diagnosis should be assessed and managed by medical and surgical specialists who are experienced in dealing with hereditary colorectal cancer syndrome families. In addition to possible genetic or other testing, initial colorectal testing should start early. In the case of FAP, a screening program that includes some form of scoping should be started at age 13. In HNPCC, periodic colorectal examination should begin no later than age 25. Additional periodic screening of the upper gastrointestinal tract in FAP family members, and of the lining of the uterus in HNPCC family members, may be recommended by the specialist. See Chapter 42 for additional detail on hereditary colorectal cancer syndromes.

6

SYMPTOMS AND SIGNS OF COLORECTAL CANCER

CHAPTER 10
SYMPTOMS OF COLORECTAL CANCER

Symptoms are the physical problems or changes that a patient notices and can describe to a doctor. The wide variety of possible symptoms includes things like weakness, pain, bleeding, a lump, and so on. If left unidentified, colorectal cancer will eventually produce symptoms.

GENERAL SYMPTOMS OF COLORECTAL CANCER

FATIGUE

If enough blood is lost from a colorectal cancer, symptoms of anemia may develop. Anemia is a state in which there are not enough oxygen-carrying red blood cells, resulting in insufficient oxygen delivery to the organs of the body. The symptoms of anemia include fatigue and lightheadedness, shortness of breath, and angina (chest pain from reduced flow of oxygen to the heart). Symptoms will initially be noticed during periods of exertion when our bodies need extra oxygen. If anemia becomes severe, tiredness may even occur when resting.

WEIGHT LOSS AND DIMINISHED APPETITE

Weight loss and diminished appetite occur late in the course of cancer growth. Almost without exception, other evidence of cancer will be present by the time the patient begins to lose weight and appetite.

SYMPTOMS FROM THE PRIMARY (ORIGINAL) SITE OF CANCER

RECTAL BLEEDING

Visible bleeding from the rectum may be a symptom of colorectal cancer and should be investigated promptly by a physician. Fortunately, most rectal bleeding is caused by benign problems and is not life-threatening. To make the distinction, however, careful review by a physician is required.

The physician can often evaluate the significance of the bleeding by asking questions about the characteristics of the blood. Bleeding from hemorrhoids is bright red. It is almost always totally painless. Bleeding from a fissure in the anus is also bright red but is usually accompanied by pain or soreness when wiping. The blood from a fissure is typically seen as streaks of bright red blood on the toilet paper. In both of these conditions, the color of the stool itself is usually normal, although there might be some blood on the surface of an otherwise normal brown stool.

Blood from a bowel cancer is painless, and is usually darker red to purple. It may be mixed in with the stool rather than merely on the surface. It may be accompanied by slime or mucus so that the blood takes on the consistency and appearance of strawberry jam. In some cases, bowel movements may consist almost entirely of this jam-like substance.

People are often very good at knowing the difference between benign rectal bleeding and bleeding originating from something more serious. When it is from a cancer, they will frequently express the opinion that this is different from any bleeding they might have had from this area in the past.

BLOATING AND CONSTIPATION

Intermittent bloating and constipation are symptoms that almost everyone experiences from time to time, but when these symptoms are persistent or increasing, they need to be investigated. Bloating and increasing constipation are relatively late symptoms of colorectal cancer. They imply that there is a growing blockage in the intestine, leading to a build-up of gas and stool above the obstruction. Surprisingly, gas and stool can get through very small openings, so these symptoms are often found late, in patients with large, advanced cancers. Such patients will also complain of an increasingly noisy or gurgling abdomen. These sounds are from the air in the bowel being moved forcibly as the intestine contracts to overcome the blockage.

CHANGE IN STOOL SHAPE OR WIDTH, OR SMALLER FREQUENT STOOLS

People will frequently express concern that their stool is narrower than usual, or an odd shape, and wonder if this could be due to a cancer. While stool narrowing can occasionally result from a large rectal cancer, the vast majority of cases of narrowed stools are from benign muscle spasms within the bowel.

Smaller, more frequent stools, especially if accompanied by blood or slime, are more worrisome. Patients with growing rectal cancers will often have more frequent bowel movements as the rectum begins to lose its capacity and becomes more regularly filled with mucus or bloody discharge from the cancer.

PAIN

Pain is not typical of colorectal cancer since the bowel itself is fairly insensitive. It is only when the cancer has penetrated through the wall of the bowel and into a more sensitive structure (such as the tailbone or muscles of the pelvis) that the person experiences pain. Thus, pain from a colorectal cancer is a late symptom and suggests an advanced cancer.

SYMPTOMS OF CANCER SPREAD

The most common site for colorectal cancer spread (metastases) is the liver. These are initially without symptoms. Growing metastases in the liver can eventually cause pain if they become large enough to stretch the surface covering of the liver. Lung metastases rarely cause symptoms unless they are very large or numerous, in which case one might expect symptoms of chest fullness, shortness of breath, cough, or pain with deep breathing. Bone metastases, as seen in prostate and other cancers, are very rare in colorectal cancer, so bone pain is almost never a sign of colorectal metastases. Very occasionally, colorectal cancer may spread to the brain, giving rise to seizures or possible psychological symptoms.

CHAPTER 11
SIGNS OF COLORECTAL CANCER

Signs of a disease are things that can be seen, heard, measured, or felt by a physician. A physician will always begin a meeting with a patient by taking a history in order to elicit symptoms of disease. He or she will then examine the patient to determine whether there are any signs of disease. Colorectal cancer may or may not provide any signs for the physician to find during an initial examination. This will depend upon how advanced the cancer is and the thoroughness of the examination.

GENERAL SIGNS THAT SOMETHING IS WRONG

Through years of experience in dealing with patients, physicians develop an ability to determine who is and who is not ill. Often, a brief visual scan is all that is required, and this can be done as the physician approaches the bedside or greets a patient in his or her office. General signs are those signs that give disease away at a glance. They include a noticeable loss of energy and vitality, a visibly depressed or quiet mood, an obvious loss of weight often most evident in the face and hands or a sallow (yellow-orange) tint to the complexion. These signs occur late in the development of the cancer, but they nonetheless may be the first sign of an underlying problem.

The cause of these general signs is poorly understood. A prominent theory is that the cancer produces proteins or other substances that interfere with normal body function and control centers, leading, for instance, to a diminished appetite. Weight loss may be due to reduced food intake in such cases, but the substances produced by the cancer may also have a direct effect on metabolism, producing weight loss greater than what could be attributed to a change in diet.

SIGNS OF THE CANCER ITSELF (AT ITS PRIMARY SITE)

The site of origin (primary site) of the cancer may be felt as a mass or lump. In the case of a low rectal cancer, the physician may be able to feel the mass when he or she examines the patient's rectum with a finger. Cancers in the upper parts of the rectum and in the colon are out of range of an examining finger, and other tests must be used to identify them (scoping, see Chapter 7). Large colon cancers may be felt by the doctor during examination of the abdomen. Rectal cancers, because they lie within the boney pelvis, can rarely be felt through the abdomen.

SIGNS THAT CANCER HAS SPREAD TO OTHER SITES

LYMPH NODE METASTASES

Colorectal cancer may spread (metastasize) through lymphatic vessels to lymph nodes or through blood vessels to other body organs. Most lymph nodes associated with the colon and rectum are positioned deep within the abdomen and cannot be felt during a physical examination. Only the very last or highest lymph node in the chain is within reach of examination. It lies behind the left collarbone close to the neck and can be felt only if it does contain cancer. This is quite a rare finding.

CANCER SPREAD THROUGH THE BLOODSTREAM
TO OTHER SITES OF THE BODY

Because blood from the colon and rectum drains directly to the liver through the portal venous system, the liver is the organ most frequently involved when colorectal cancer spreads through the blood stream. Single cancer cells or clumps of cancer cells loose in the bloodstream lodge in the liver and begin growing into larger masses (metastases.) Depending on the size of the metastases, their location within the liver, the experience of the examining physician, and the thickness of the abdominal wall (Figure 13), liver metastases may or may not be felt when present.

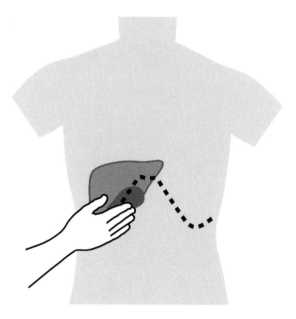

Figure 13. *Feeling for a liver metastasis.*

CANCER THAT HAS SPREAD TO THE ABDOMINAL CAVITY

In advanced cases of colorectal cancer in which the cancer has penetrated through the bowel wall and is exposed on the surface of the bowel within the abdomen, malignant cells may fall off the cancer and spread within the abdominal cavity. They may settle in the pelvis and grow outside of the colon, forming lumps in the pelvis or on the membrane (peritoneum) that lines the abdominal cavity. If these lumps are present and growing in the pelvis, they can sometimes be felt by an experienced physician during rectal examination.

DIAGNOSIS OF COLORECTAL CANCER

7

When the physician has assessed the patient's symptoms and signs, there may be enough evidence to warrant testing to confirm or rule out the diagnosis of cancer. This will include some method of viewing the colon, either by direct viewing through a scope, or by an X-ray called a *barium enema* (see Chapter 7 for details). A sample of tissue (biopsy) is needed in order to confirm the diagnosis. Since scope tests are the most accurate way of assessing the colon and they allow for biopsies, they are usually preferred to a barium enema if cancer is suspected.

DIRECT VIEWING SCOPES

A variety of instruments is available for looking into the bowel. Collectively, these instruments are called *endoscopes*. "Endo" means inside. These instruments may be rigid or flexible, varying in length from just a few centimeters to 160 cm (63 inches).

RIGID SIGMOIDOSCOPE

A rigid sigmoidoscope measures 25 cm in length and 1.9 cm in width (10 inches by $^1/_2$ inch) and is equipped with a light to permit the doctor to look down the bore of the instrument into the rectum (see Chapter 7 for more detail).

FLEXIBLE SIGMOIDOSCOPE

A flexible sigmoidoscope is 60 cm (24 inches) long. This permits the physician to examine further up the bowel, often reaching the area of the mid or upper descending colon. Since the colon and rectum may measure up to 160 cm (63 inches), flexible sigmoidoscopes are too short to assess the entire colon (see Chapter 7 for more detail).

COLONOSCOPE

The colonoscope is a 160 cm (63 inch) flexible instrument that can assess the entire colon and rectum. Of all the available diagnostic tools for the colon, colonoscopy provides the highest level of accuracy (see Chapter 7 for more detail). Figure k in the color section shows a typical colorectal cancer as seen with a colonoscope.

BARIUM ENEMA

A barium enema is an X-ray that permits examination of the colon and rectum. It is not as accurate as colonoscopy and one cannot take biopsies or remove a polyp during a barium enema (see Chapter 7 for additional information).

BIOPSY

When a lump or mass is found, an experienced physician can often tell from its appearance whether it is a cancer. However, the pathologist makes the final diagnosis by viewing a sample of the mass under the microscope. The physician obtains a sample of the mass for the pathologist to examine. The sample is called a *biopsy*. A biopsy is taken through one of the endoscopes (Figure c(ii), color section). Most biopsies are tiny, often no more than a millimeter or two in diameter ($^1/_8$ inch), but still contain thousands of cells for the pathologist to examine. The patient should not experience any pain when the biopsy is being taken.

QUESTIONS

IF THE BARIUM ENEMA SUGGESTS A CANCER, IS A BIOPSY NECESSARY BEFORE SURGERY?

In some cases, a barium enema result may be so suggestive of cancer that the surgeon decides to go ahead and operate to remove a portion of bowel without first obtaining a biopsy confirming the diagnosis. While this usually results in the correct treatment, it is not recommended unless a preliminary biopsy cannot be obtained. Unlike direct viewing provided by an endoscope, the barium enema shows only shadows of what may be in the bowel. Sometimes an intestinal spasm may look so much like the shadow of a cancer that the physician mistakenly interprets it as being a cancer. There have been cases in which this has led to unnecessary major surgery where nothing whatsoever was found. Unless there are overwhelming reasons to forego direct endoscopic viewing and biopsy, a barium enema should not be relied upon as the sole means of diagnosis. If it is at all possible to obtain, a biopsy-proven diagnosis is always preferred.

WHAT IF THE BIOPSY OF A SUSPICIOUS MASS COMES BACK AS NORMAL?

As a general principle, a biopsy of a suspicious area that is reported as normal should not be taken at face value. If surgeons see what appears to be a cancer through a colonoscope and takes a biopsy of it, they expect the pathologist to agree with their visual interpretation. If the pathologist claims the tissue is benign (that is, normal), it may mean that the surgeon missed the cancerous part of the mass with his or her biopsy. The cancer may be covered in benign inflamed tissue (Figure 14) or the colonoscopist may have missed the important area completely. The pathologist can only report on what he or she is given. If there is a discrepancy, a second set of biopsies may be in order.

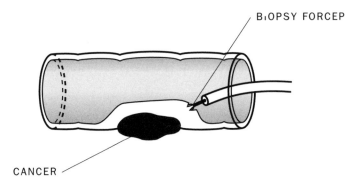

Figure 14. *A small biopsy forcep may miss a cancer. A cancer may still be present when the biopsy is normal.*

WHAT IS STAGING?

Once the diagnosis of colorectal cancer is made, other tests are needed to determine how far the cancer has spread. This is called *staging* a cancer. The treatment and outlook for colorectal cancer depends, to a large extent, on its stage.

A cancer that is small and confined to its primary (original) site at the time of diagnosis is an *early stage* cancer, likely to be cured with surgery alone. A cancer that has spread to other parts of the body, or has penetrated very deeply, is a *late stage* (advanced) cancer, and surgery alone might not cure the disease. Other treatments such as chemotherapy or radiation therapy may be required. Staging represents the best attempt to determine the degree of cancer spread. In some cases, it may not be entirely accurate since at any time a few tiny cancer cells may be on the move in numbers too small to be detected by any staging test.

Staging is begun once the diagnosis of cancer is made because initial treatment will be based upon this staging information. After surgery, the information gained during the operation and the pathologist's assessment of the removed specimen provide additional information to complete the staging process.

THE STAGING TESTS

ALKALINE PHOSPHATASE BLOOD TEST

Alkaline phosphatase is an enzyme produced by the bile ducts of the liver. When the bile ducts become blocked by deposits of cancer, alkaline phosphatase accumulates within the ducts and enters the bloodstream. A blood sample showing an elevated level of alkaline phosphatase suggests liver metastases (that is, cancer that has spread to the liver). The presence or absence of liver metastases should be confirmed by other tests as well.

CARCINOEMBRYONIC ANTIGEN (CEA) BLOOD TEST

Some colorectal cancers produce a protein called *carcinoembryonic antigen* (*CEA*) that circulates in the blood. The amount of CEA circulating is directly related to the amount of cancer that is present. Many colorectal cancer patients have normal CEA levels when the cancer is first identified, suggesting small, localized cancers. Elevations during the course of treatment and recovery usually signal the development of an increasing amount of cancer, suggesting metastases or recurrence. If the CEA is elevated when a colorectal cancer patient is first diagnosed, it may mean that the cancer is very large, or that metastases already exist.

COLONOSCOPY

If it has not already been done, a colonoscopy should be performed to rule out other problems within the colon. A small percentage of patients (3%) with one identified colorectal cancer will have a second cancer at the same time, while 15% will have polyps elsewhere in the colon.

CHEST X-RAY

Chest X-rays permit a radiologist to determine whether there is any obvious spread of the colorectal cancer to the lungs (Figure l, color section). Lung metastases in colorectal cancer are not usually seen until the cancer is advanced. Since the liver is the most common site of metastases from colorectal cancer, lung metastases suggest that cancer is probably present in the liver as well.

ABDOMINAL ULTRASOUND

Ultrasound examinations use sound waves to outline the structures within the body. A radiologist moves a special hand-held sound wave generator and receiver across the abdomen (Figure m, color section). As the sound waves penetrate the abdomen, the various abdominal organs reflect them back to the receiver. The reflected waves are processed electronically to produce a picture of the abdominal contents on a computer screen. Ultrasound detects liver metastases very accurately. Ultrasound is not normally effective for detecting a colon or rectal cancer primary site (in the bowel) unless the cancer is very large.

ENDORECTAL ULTRASOUND

Endorectal ultrasound is an ultrasound examination of the rectum and adjacent tissues that is performed by inserting a special ultrasound probe through the anus and into the low rectum (Figure n(i), color section). Endorectal ultrasound is useful for staging rectal cancer. Endorectal (which means inside the rectum) ultrasound can assess the depth that a rectal cancer penetrates into the wall of the rectum (Figure n(ii) and (iii), color section). It can also indicate whether there are any adjacent lymph nodes that may be enlarged—a sign of possible lymph node metastases. The drawbacks of endorectal ultrasound are that it can only identify rectal cancers within the 10 to 13 cm (four to five inch) range of the probe, it is dependant upon the ultrasound operator's expertise, and it cannot be used on very large or low cancers. Also, it doesn't precisely show the membrane (mesorectal fascia) that surrounds the rectum and its lymph nodes. Determining whether a rectal cancer has penetrated this membrane is important staging information. MRI, discussed on the next page, is the superior test for viewing the surrounding membrane.

CT SCAN

The *CT scan* (also CAT scan, computerized axial tomography) is a sophisticated computerized X-ray that produces a series of slice-through views of the patient's body. The patient is placed on a special automated stretcher that moves slowly through a large circular device or ring (Figure o(i), color section). The ring consists of a circle of X-ray machines that take X-rays simultaneously. A computer combines the data into an image of what one would see if the body had been sliced across from one side to the other (Figure 15 and Figure o(ii), color section). The CT scan can be useful to determine the spread of cancer in the abdomen by detecting enlarged lymph nodes and metastases.

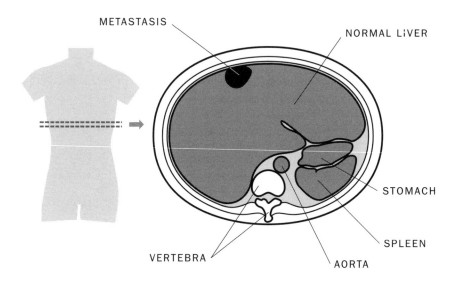

Figure 15. *CT section. Colon cancer metastasis seen within the liver.*

MRI

The *MRI* (magnetic resonance imaging) is a very high-tech machine that uses magnetic fields to provide images of tissue. The patient lies within a chamber in which magnetic field changes are produced, and the body's response to these magnetic changes is recorded and processed into an image that looks almost three-dimensional. The MRI is particularly useful in the local staging of rectal cancer as it shows, in great detail, the mesorectal membrane surrounding the fat and lymph nodes of the rectum. The MRI can identify penetration through the membrane by a rectal cancer.

TYPICAL PRE-TREATMENT STAGING PROTOCOLS

COLON CANCER

Once a colon cancer has been found, a full colonoscopy is done to ensure there are no other lesions in the colon. Typically, alkaline phosphatase and CEA blood tests will be obtained, along with a chest X-ray and either an abdominal ultrasound or a CT scan of the abdomen. The main purpose of the abdominal ultrasound or CT scan is to alert the surgeon to the possible presence of liver metastases, which he or she may wish to be prepared for at the time of surgery.

RECTAL CANCER

Staging for rectal cancer is more sophisticated than for colon cancer since the treatment for rectal cancer has greater variations than colon cancer treatment. In addition to the blood tests (alkaline phosphatase and CEA), colonoscopy, chest X-ray, and either abdominal ultrasound or abdominal CT scan, careful assessment of the rectal area is done. That assessment starts with the examiner's finger in the rectum. If the cancer is freely mobile in the soft tissues of the pelvis, it means that it has likely not penetrated the mesorectal fascia (membrane), and endorectal ultrasound is a good method of determining its depth. If, however, the tumor is large, very low, or seems tethered to surrounding tissues, an MRI is a better choice for assessing the rectum, since tethering indicates that the cancer has likely penetrated through the mesorectal fascia into surrounding tissues of the pelvis. The MRI is excellent for viewing these deeper penetrations, whereas the endorectal ultrasound cannot show this depth.

TWO

WHAT ARE MY OPTIONS NOW THAT I HAVE
A DIAGNOSIS OF COLORECTAL CANCER?

TREATMENT PLANNING

8

CHAPTER 14
AN OVERVIEW OF COLORECTAL
CANCER TREATMENT

THE CANCER STAGE GUIDES TREATMENT

Whether surgery is performed at all, the type of operation used, and whether chemotherapy or radiation is given in addition to surgery all depend upon the stage of the cancer. Be sure to ask your doctor to explain the stage of your cancer so you can understand how your treatment will be planned.

SURGERY THROUGH THE ABDOMEN IS THE MAINSTAY OF TREATMENT

In most cases, the treatment for colorectal cancer is surgery. In some situations, when the cancers are found very early and are still quite small, the surgery may be fairly limited, as in the case of a small malignant polyp that just needs to be removed with a colonoscope, or the rare small rectal cancer that may simply be excised through the anus. But in most patients, colorectal cancer is more advanced than this when it is diagnosed, so that these simple treatments are not appropriate. Instead, most patients will require one of the more traditional operations in which the cancerous segment of the colon or rectum is removed through an incision in the abdomen.

RADIATION THERAPY AND CHEMOTHERAPY MAY BE USED TO ENHANCE THE EFFECT OF SURGERY

PREOPERATIVE THERAPY

In some cases, surgery for rectal cancer may be more successful if radiotherapy to the rectum is given prior to the operation. It is generally given if staging tests determine that the rectal cancer is deeply penetrating. Colon cancer patients, on the other hand, are not typically given preoperative radiotherapy.

POSTOPERATIVE THERAPY

After surgery, the doctors have the advantage of knowing more about the cancer than they did prior to surgery. They have the information that the surgeon discovered during the operation such as how difficult the cancer was to remove and whether there were any unsuspected metastases seen. In addition, the pathologist now has a chance to look carefully at the entire removed cancer, not just the small preoperative biopsy. An accurate assessment of the lymph nodes and the cancer's depth of penetration can be made. After rectal cancer surgery, depending upon this information from the specimen, chemotherapy, and/or radiotherapy may be given postoperatively to enhance the possible cure if the cancer was deeply penetrating or the specimen shows positive lymph nodes. After colon cancer surgery, chemotherapy, but rarely radiotherapy, may be given if the lymph nodes are found to be positive for cancer.

A PERMANENT COLOSTOMY IS NOT NECESSARY IN MOST CASES

The vast majority of patients who undergo surgery for colorectal cancer do not end up with a colostomy (opening on the abdominal wall for stool). Generally, the bowel will be put back together after the cancerous segment is removed, so that bowel movements will be passed in the usual way. Only when the cancer is very low in the rectum (within the reach of the physician's examining finger) does the possibility of a permanent colostomy arise.

CHAPTER 15
THE STAGES OF COLORECTAL CANCER

There is more than one system of terminology designed to describe colorectal cancer stage. The most commonly used systems are the TNM system, the Dukes system, and the Astler-Coller system. This book will focus on the *TNM system*, which is the most widely used at major cancer centers. The TNM system uses information about a patient's tumor (T), lymph nodes (N), and the presence or absence of metastases (M) to determine the stage of that patient's colorectal cancer. The stage is listed as Roman numerals I to IV.

T CATEGORIES FOR TNM STAGING SYSTEM

T categories represent different depths of the tumor's (cancer's) penetration. The deeper the layer of intestine that the tumor has penetrated, the greater the T category of that tumor. To best understand this, some knowledge of the intestine layers is helpful (Figure 16).

The layers of the intestine, from the inside to the outside, are the lining (*mucosa*), the fibrous tissue beneath this layer (*submucosa*), the thick muscle layer of the bowel wall (*muscularis propria*) and the thin outermost layer (subserosa and *serosa*). An additional layer of importance in rectal cancer is the membrane (*mesorectal fascia*) that surrounds the rectum and the lymph nodes behind it.

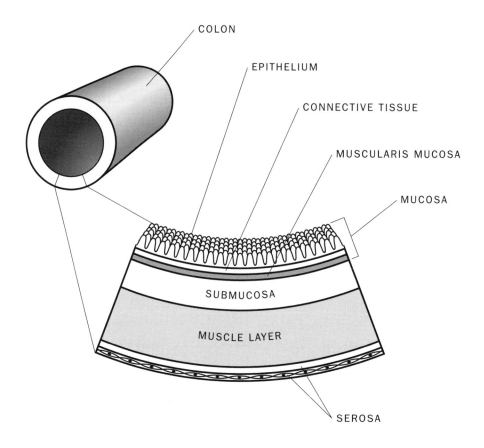

COLON

EPITHELIUM

CONNECTIVE TISSUE

MUSCULARIS MUCOSA

MUCOSA

SUBMUCOSA

MUSCLE LAYER

SEROSA

Figure 16. *The layers of the intestine wall.*

TIS: The cancer is in the earliest stage, known as *carcinoma-in-situ* or *intramucosal carcinoma*. It has not grown beyond the mucosa (inner layer) of the colon or rectum.

T1: The cancer has grown through the mucosa and extends into the submucosa.

T2: The cancer has grown through the submucosa and extends into the thick muscle layer (muscularis propria).

T3: The cancer has grown completely through the thick muscle layer but not into adjacent organs.

T4: The cancer has grown right through the wall of the colon or rectum into nearby tissues or organs.

N CATEGORIES FOR TNM STAGING SYSTEM

N categories indicate whether the cancer has spread to nearby lymph nodes and, if so, how many lymph nodes are involved.

NX: No description of lymph node involvement is possible because of incomplete information.

N0: No examined lymph nodes contain cancer.

N1: Cancer cells found in one to three regional (nearby) lymph nodes.

N2: Cancer cells found in four or more regional lymph nodes.

M CATEGORIES FOR TNM STAGING SYSTEM

M categories indicate whether or not the cancer has spread to distant organs, such as the liver, lungs.

M0: No distant spread has been found.

M1: Distant spread has been found.

GROUPING THE TNM INFORMATION INTO STAGES

Once a patient's T, N, and M categories have been determined, usually after surgery, this information is combined in a process called stage grouping to determine the stage, expressed in Roman numerals from stage I (the least advanced stage) to stage IV (the most advanced stage). The following guide illustrates how TNM categories are grouped together into stages (see Figure 17):

STAGE 0: TIS, N0, M0: The cancer is in the earliest stage. It has not grown beyond the inner layer (mucosa) of the colon or rectum. This stage is also known as carcinoma in situ or intramucosal carcinoma.

STAGE I: T1, N0, M0, OR T2, N0, M0: The cancer has grown through the mucosa into the submucosa or it may also have grown into the thick muscle layer, but it has not spread into the nearby lymph nodes and there are no metastases.

STAGE IIA: T3, N0, M0: The cancer has grown through the thick muscle layer but is still contained by the outermost layers, serosa or mesorectal fascia, and has not spread to the lymph nodes or distant sites.

STAGE IIB: T4, N0, M0: The cancer has grown through the wall of the bowel and the outermost layers and into nearby tissues or organs. It has not spread to the lymph nodes or distant sites.

STAGE IIIA: T1 OR T2, N1, M0: The cancer has grown through the mucosa into the submucosa or it may also have grown into the thick muscle layer, and it has spread to one to three nearby lymph nodes but no distant sites.

STAGE IIIB: T3 OR T4, N1, M0: The cancer has grown through the wall of the colon or rectum or into other nearby tissues or organs and has spread to one to three nearby lymph nodes but no distant sites.

STAGE IIIC: ANY T, N2, M0: The cancer may be any T but has spread to four or more nearby lymph nodes but no distant sites.

STAGE IV: ANY T, ANY N, M1: The cancer can be any T, any N, but has spread to distant sites such as the liver, lung, peritoneum (the membrane lining the abdominal cavity), or ovary.

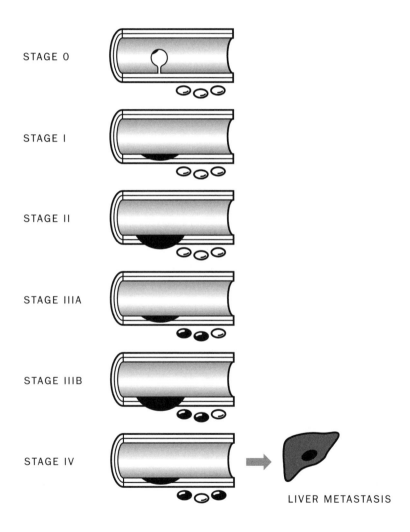

Figure 17. *Cancer stages.*

USING TNM STAGES AS A GUIDELINE TO TREATMENT

The following are the general guidelines for treating colorectal cancer based upon TNM stage.

STAGE 0

This is usually a polyp. Treatment consists of removal of the polyp only.

STAGE I

Surgical removal of that part of the bowel only.

STAGE II

Surgical removal of that part of the bowel. Possible preoperative radiation if it is a rectal cancer. Possible chemotherapy postoperatively for either rectal or colon cancer.

STAGE III

Surgical removal of that part of the bowel, possible preoperative radiation if it is a rectal cancer. Chemotherapy postoperatively for either rectal or colon cancer. Possible postoperative radiotherapy if rectal cancer and radiotherapy was not given prior to surgery.

STAGE IV

Surgical removal of the colon or rectal cancer if the patient is in reasonable condition. Possible removal of metastases. Possible chemotherapy. In some very advanced cases, the cancer may not be removed if the patient is very frail and not expected to live long.

The above guidelines are meant as an overview only. Cancer treatment and treatment related to stage will be discussed in more depth in Sections 9, 10, and 13.

CHAPTER 16
STRATEGIES FOR NAVIGATING THE CANCER CARE SYSTEM

The treatment of cancer involves many different health care providers. Although most patients assume that these people work as part of a well-coordinated team, unfortunately, this is often not the case. Even though each professional is a qualified specialist in her or his field, each may work in relative isolation from the other team members.

FIND A HELPER IF YOU CAN

In most situations, there is no single medical person who functions in the role of case manager to coordinate a patient's medical files and his or her passage through the treatment system. Many patients expect that their family physician will take on this role, but it is not a responsibility that many family physicians can assume. Not all medical reports are automatically forwarded to the family physician and those that are may be slow in arriving. The average family physician will have only a few patients with a new cancer diagnosis each year, so they may not feel well-equipped to handle the details of the multiple treatment options.

As a result, many patients find that they need someone, other than themselves, to act as a navigator or case manager to help them sift, organize, integrate, and keep track of all the information, advice, and appointments they encounter. While it might seem that patients would make the best case managers since they know the most about their history and any special health problems, most cancer treatments subject the patient to a high degree of physical and psychological strain. Thus, the addition of case-management responsibilities to this load creates a huge additional burden. Typically, the person who takes on this role is a spouse, partner, relative, or close friend. No medical background is necessary, although it helps. The most important thing is a willingness to devote the time and attention needed to help the patient.

Listed below are some examples of the duties a case manager might undertake (with the patient's consent):

- Keeping a binder with copies of all test results and procedures.
- Keeping a written record of all instructions regarding prescriptions.
- Keeping track of all tests requested by each physician. Often, during the course of treatments, two physicians who are treating the patient at the same time will ask for the same test to be done. The case manager can offer the test results (or at least mention their existence) to the second physician. This saves the patient from having to undergo the procedure again, and the medical system from the cost of a duplicate test.
- Informing each new health care provider about any special characteristics or problems that the patient has.
  - A simple example: if the patient normally has low blood pressure, this is helpful information for each health care provider to know as they prepare to take one of the dozens of blood pressure readings that the patient will undergo over the course of treatments.
  - A more significant example: if it is difficult to draw blood from the patient, the case manager can inform the technician beforehand. This

may alter the technician's approach or procedure and could save the patient from having extra punctures in his or her arm from second tries.

- A serious example: if the patient has any unusual reaction to anesthesia, this information should be given to the anesthetist. This is especially important if operations are performed in different hospitals, since information about previous anesthetic problems is not necessarily passed between medical teams.

To be most helpful, the case manager needs to accompany the patient to most, if not all, appointments, tests, and procedures. Almost all health care providers will allow the case manager to stay with the patient. The patient might phrase the request: "I would like John to stay with me for this test/treatment. Would this be all right?" You may be surprised to find that this arrangement can even extend to being allowed to stay in the room during minor surgery.

HELPFUL QUESTIONS TO ASK ABOUT DRUG OR OTHER THERAPY

When the patient has been prescribed a new drug or treatment as part of his or her cancer care, the case manager should ask specific questions to the physician, pharmacist, or nurse before starting the drug. These questions should also be asked to an alternative health care practitioner, such as a naturopath, who has prescribed alternative therapies such as herbal remedies or vitamins.

1. Why is this drug or treatment being prescribed?
2. What is the goal of the therapy? Is it for cure? Is it to slow disease? Is it to relieve symptoms?
3. Is this a standard or a new therapy? What is the evidence for using this particular protocol?
4. How do we know if the drug or treatment is working? If there is recurrent disease will the cancer disappear or stop growing, or will the patient just

feel better? What happens if the drug or treatment doesn't work? Should the drug be stopped or the dose increased? What happens if it still doesn't work when the dose is increased? Are there other treatment options?

5. When can we tell if treatment is working? If it works, will it be continued, and for how long?

6. What are the potential harmful effects? How should we recognize and manage them?

7. Who should we call if there are problems or if we have more questions?

A WORD ABOUT THE INTERNET

Many patients and their case managers will have access to the Internet for retrieving information about cancer. The Internet is a mixed blessing in that it contains almost as much potentially harmful information as it does helpful information. Ask your physician for names of websites that he or she feels are credible and be sure to check back with the information you find to ensure that it is relevant to your problem and treatment program.

HELPFUL HINTS FOR THE CASE MANAGER

▶ Take a notebook and a tape recorder to all appointments. (Alert the physician before using the tape recorder.)

▶ Ask for copies of all medical and pathology reports. This is a patient's right under freedom-of-information laws in most places. This information allows you to double-check that new reports do not contradict previous reports. They also give you a better understanding of what is happening.

▶ Speak up when you are becoming frustrated with information overload or conflicting information. If necessary, put your concerns in writing (tactfully and positively).

▶ Carry a cell phone or pager if you can't be easily reached. Either can be rented for several months.

▶ Understand that patient medical files are used to record procedures and test results. They might not record all the instructions or explanations given by each health care provider. Each new health care provider can only guess at what has been explained before.

▶ Remember that patient medical files are not routinely passed from one health care facility to another unless the patient or physician requests specific information.

▶ If possible, secure the support of a physician who is a friend or family member and who is not directly involved in the patient's care. This person can be a valuable source of general medical knowledge, including insights into how the system works.

▶ Encourage the patient to have a good relationship with his or her family physician. Although specialists direct most of the cancer-specific treatments, it is the family physician who maintains contact with the patient after the cancer treatments are completed.

▶ Often, when specialists receive test results, especially negative results (that is, results are normal), they are not passed on until the next scheduled appointment. This is a good time to call upon the family physician (to whom test results are usually forwarded) for an earlier interpretation of the results. Sometimes the family physician doesn't receive these results either, but it's worth asking.

▶ Before the patient sees a specialist such as a surgeon or oncologist, fax any questions you have first. Because of their busy schedules, they may find it helpful to receive the questions in writing and in advance of the appointment.

▶ Maintain a calm, caring presence for the sake of the patient and yourself.

▶ Think of ways to reduce the patient's stress. For example, suggest that call display on the phone would allow the patient to answer only the calls he or she chooses while you could respond to the rest when time is available.

- ► Remember that your job is not to become a medical expert, but an expert on what has happened (treatments, patient moods, test results, etc.) in relation to your relative or friend.

- ► Understand that almost every health care provider is a skilled expert, but is probably overworked, with more than the optimal number of patients. They are doing their best and your goal is to help them achieve this.

- ► Express your appreciation when the health care provider does something praiseworthy.

- ► Allow your friends and relatives to help you so that you can take care of yourself also. It is essential that you do not burn out. (Some areas have caregiver support groups. Ask at the hospital about this if you are interested.)

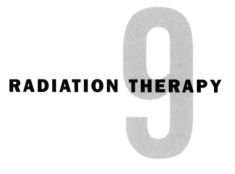

RADIATION THERAPY

CHAPTER 17
WHAT IS RADIATION THERAPY
AND HOW IS IT GIVEN?

Radiation therapy, also called *radiotherapy*, is the use of high-energy rays to kill cancer cells. A physician who specializes in treating cancer patients with radiation is called a *radiation oncologist*. Radiation works by damaging the cells so that they eventually die. Radiation will damage any type of cell, either normal or cancerous, that lies in the path of the beam. Therefore, great care must be taken to aim the beam only at the part of the body that needs treatment and avoid exposing healthy tissue to radiation as much as possible.

Fortunately, normal cells repair themselves from radiation damage more completely than cancer cells do. So, by giving the radiation in a series of small treatments, usually once a day, normal cells have a chance to recover between treatments while the cancer cells die. However, when high dose radiotherapy is used to treat a cancer, there is inevitably some damage to the surrounding tissue. The art of radiotherapy is to maximize the chance of curing the cancer while at the same time limiting the damage to normal tissue so that it is below the level at which it causes symptoms.

WHEN IS RADIATION GIVEN?

Radiation therapy is used to help prevent recurrence or progression of cancer in a specific part of the body, for example the rectum or adjacent pelvis. Given before or after rectal surgery, radiation is directed to the pelvis to kill any cancer cells that may not be removed by the surgery.

It can also be used to treat metastatic cancer in a particular part of the body. For instance, if rectal cancer has spread to a bony part of the spine and causes pain, radiation to the affected area will kill many of the cancer cells there and relieve the pain.

The benefits and side effects of radiation therapy are generally restricted to the area being treated, except for fatigue, which is a common side effect of any radiation therapy.

THE PROCEDURE FOR GETTING RADIOTHERAPY

The process can be considered in three steps:

1. Deciding whether radiotherapy should be given.
2. Planning how the radiotherapy should be given.
3. Receiving the daily radiotherapy treatment.

THE TREATMENT DECISION

You make the decision to proceed with radiotherapy in consultation with a radiation oncologist (a specialist in radiation therapy). The issues to consider are described in the next chapter.

THE PLANNING SESSION

The purpose of the planning session is to plan exactly how the radiotherapy machine is to be aimed, given your individual size and body shape, and the part of the body that requires treatment. The area to be treated is identified by using a machine called a simulator. The simulator may be a CT scanner or a low energy X-ray machine. Either machine can produce images that the radiation oncologist needs to identify the area requiring treatment. Once this area is identified, the treatment planning unit staff and the radiation oncologist work together to find the best combination of radiation beams to treat the area. The planning session usually takes about half an hour.

Very specific information is recorded during the planning session so that the X-ray machine can be accurately repositioned each time you arrive for a treatment. Initially, temporary lines are drawn on the skin to assist in targeting the tumor site. These temporary lines may be replaced by small, permanent ink dots (tattoos) the size of a small freckle. They are usually placed at the centre or corner of the treatment area. One advantage of permanent tattoos is that they help avoid the mistake of repeating treatment to the same area if radiation is considered sometime in the future.

TREATMENT SESSIONS

The amount of radiation and number of daily visits is determined by how much tissue needs treatment, the location and whether the goal is to prevent recurrence or to relieve symptoms caused by cancer. If it is to prevent cancer from coming back, the treatment consists of four to six weeks of daily treatments. However, in some circumstances, a one week course of treatment is given before surgery. When the goal is symptom relief only, the length of the course of radiation treatment may vary from one to 15 or more daily treatments depending on the circumstances.

WHAT HAPPENS DURING RADIATION TREATMENT?

Radiation treatments are painless. In fact, when the machine is on, the only thing you'll notice is a slight whirring sound. Treatments may be given from several angles each day to make sure that the entire targeted area gets treated.

For each visit, you will be in the treatment room for about 10 to 20 minutes. The radiation therapist spends most of this time carefully adjusting the X-ray machine so that it is positioned correctly. During a typical session, the machine is turned on for only one to five minutes for each area being treated on a given day.

HOW MUCH RADIATION IS GIVEN DURING RADIOTHERAPY?

The radiation dose delivered is limited by what the normal tissues in the treated area can tolerate. The basic unit of radiation dose is called a *Gray*. The amount of radiation received during a chest X-ray is approximately 0.005 Gray. In contrast, the total dose typically used to treat the rectal area during cancer therapy ranges from 25 Gray (divided into five doses over one week) to 45 and up to 60 Gray (given daily over five to six-and-a-half weeks).

BRACHYTHERAPY—ANOTHER WAY TO GIVE RADIATION

With *brachytherapy*, instead of using a machine that sends out an X-ray beam, a tiny piece of radioactive material is implanted directly into a tumor or placed immediately alongside it. Radioactive iridium is the substance most often used, but other materials such as radioactive gold and cesium are also employed.

To give brachytherapy, local or general anesthetic is used and hollow tubes are inserted into the chosen area and stitched into place. This is called an implant. Later, on the hospital ward, the doctor or technician places the radioactive iridium into the tubes, either by hand or by a remote-control device. Depending on the radioactive material used and the best way to use it, the radiation material may either be left in place continuously or inserted into the implant tubes once or twice a day for several days.

When the radioactive material is actually in place, the hospital room is considered to be radioactive and visitors are restricted. With intermittent treatment, since the tubes themselves are not radioactive, visitors are allowed between treatments.

When the radioactive material is placed alongside the tumor, for example by placing the material in a special applicator in the rectal cavity, less sedation is usually needed and a general anesthetic is rarely necessary.

CAN RADIATION BE REPEATED AT SOME TIME IN THE FUTURE?

When giving radiotherapy to a part of the body, the idea is to maximize the killing effect on the cancer while staying within safe limits in normal surrounding tissues. The maximum dose that can be given is usually the most that the normal tissues surrounding the tumor can tolerate. This dose will cause some permanent damage to these normal tissues, although this doesn't usually produce noticeable symptoms. However, if an area has been given maximum radiation in the past, full dose re-treatment of that area can't be given safely due to tissue damage that remains. Occasionally, though, the area can be re-treated to a lower dose if cancer re-growth occurs and is causing symptoms. If an entirely new area of the body develops problems from cancer, full dose treatment can be considered. In palliative treatments (that is, treatment meant to relieve symptoms, not cure the disease), a lower dose of radiation is needed and treatment to the same area can often be repeated.

CHAPTER 18
WHO BENEFITS FROM RADIATION THERAPY?

RADIOTHERAPY HELPS SOME PATIENTS WITH COLON CANCER

Radiation therapy is used only occasionally to treat patients with colon cancer because the surgeon can usually remove the cancer completely. Risk of recurrence in the area surrounding the tumor is so low that the addition of radiation therapy is of little benefit. As well, radiation directed at the abdomen can cause damage to the surrounding organs. So, given the risks and the minimal benefit, radiation to the abdomen in cases of colon cancer is not done very often.

However, some colon cancers are considered particularly high risk for recurrence, and so radiation may be considered. Such cases might include the colon cancer that grows all the way through the wall of the colon, becoming attached to the abdominal wall or another abdominal structure. In this situation radiotherapy may be given to the area where it is thought that microscopic cancer cells may have been left behind at surgery.

The other situation in which radiation is used for patients with colon cancer is to treat metastatic disease in other organs, particularly if the metastases are causing pain. More detail is given in the section on palliative radiotherapy for rectal cancer at the end of this chapter.

RADIOTHERAPY HELPS MANY PATIENTS WITH RECTAL CANCER

Radiotherapy is used much more often for patients with rectal cancer than for those with colon cancer. This is because rectal cancers are more likely to recur in the local area (the pelvis) after apparently successful surgery, particularly if the cancer is in the mid or low rectum. In addition, it is fairly safe to give radiation to the rectum since it lies below the rest of the bowel within the bony pelvis. Thus, radiation beams directed at the rectum are unlikely to injure the other, normal parts of the intestine.

There are three main situations when radiation therapy is used for patients with rectal cancer:

- ‣ Before or after surgery for rectal cancer to make the operation easier and more complete, to reduce the extent of the operation, and to reduce the risk of recurrence.

- ‣ As the only treatment when either the rectal cancer cannot be removed or the patient is not well enough to withstand an operation.

- ‣ To relieve symptoms of rectal cancer that has spread to the pelvis or elsewhere.

BEFORE OR AFTER SURGERY FOR RECTAL CANCER

The risk of rectal cancer recurrence after surgery is highest when the tumor has invaded all the way through the rectal wall or spread to the lymph nodes in the pelvis. Radiotherapy (given either on its own or in conjunction with chemotherapy) reduces the risk of recurrence compared to surgery alone for more advanced cancers.

Radiation treatment may be given either before surgery (*preoperative radiation*, sometimes called *neoadjuvant radiation*) or after surgery (*postoperative radiation*, sometimes called *adjuvant radiation*). The advantage of giving it after surgery is that all of the staging information from the pathology report is available, making the decision to give additional treatment better informed. On the other hand, it appears that preoperative treatment is slightly more effective and may cause fewer side effects than postoperative treatment. Modern diagnostic techniques such as MRI (magnetic resonance imaging) and endorectal ultrasound scans may provide the necessary staging information with a high degree of accuracy before an operation. This can identify the patients who are most likely to benefit from preoperative radiotherapy.

Preoperative (neoadjuvant) radiotherapy for rectal cancer

There are two main approaches to giving preoperative radiotherapy. The first is called *short course preoperative radiotherapy*. It is only used for cancers that appear as though they will be fairly easy to remove. The second approach is called *long course preoperative radiotherapy*. This is used when the cancer is very large, or is attached to adjacent tissue, causing the surgeon concerns that he or she might not be able to get it out during the operation. Long course preoperative radiotherapy may make a large cancer smaller and less tethered to surrounding tissues, so that it can be removed more easily and completely during surgery.

Short course preoperative radiotherapy consists of five days of treatment, with surgery to follow within the next week. This type of treatment aims to reduce the risk of recurrence by killing any cancer cells that may not be removed by surgery. Because the surgery follows very soon after the radiotherapy, there is no time for the tumor to shrink, so the type of operation to be performed is not changed.

Preoperative radiotherapy is most effective for tumors in the lower two-thirds of the rectum. In these cases, preoperative radiotherapy reduces the risk of recurrence of more advanced tumors by over 50% compared to surgery without radiation. No chemotherapy is given with this treatment, although it may be given postoperatively depending upon what is found at surgery and what the pathologist finds when examining the removed specimen.

Long course preoperative radiotherapy usually lasts four or five weeks. Chemotherapy is usually given at the same time. Then surgery follows four to eight weeks after the radiotherapy is completed. By this time, the side effects of the radiation, such as inflammation of the tissues in the pelvis, have subsided. It is also hoped that by this time, the cancer will be smaller and more easily removed. For cancers low in the rectum and close to the anus that might require removal of the anus and permanent colostomy, long course preoperative radiation may shrink the cancer enough to allow the surgeon to remove it and still save the anus.

Postoperative (adjuvant) radiotherapy for rectal cancer

This is very similar to the long course preoperative schedule. Giving chemotherapy with the radiation is more effective than giving either alone. The course may be lengthened and the dose increased if the doctors believe that the surgery hasn't removed all of the cancer from the pelvis.

AS THE ONLY TREATMENT WHEN EITHER THE RECTAL CANCER CAN'T BE REMOVED OR THE PATIENT IS NOT WELL ENOUGH TO WITHSTAND AN OPERATION

Although it is less effective than surgery, radiotherapy without surgery has a role in some situations. If possible, a schedule of combined chemotherapy and radiation similar to the long course treatments described above should be given. However, some patients with medical conditions that make the risk of surgery unacceptably high also face an increased risk of severe chemotherapy side effects. For these patients, radiotherapy may have to be given without chemotherapy. In such cases, a one to three week course of high dose radiotherapy to the pelvis often provides relief of symptoms caused by advanced tumors, such as pelvic pain, bleeding, or mucous discharge.

TO RELIEVE SYMPTOMS OF ADVANCED RECTAL OR COLON CANCER CAUSED BY METASTASES IN THE PELVIS OR ELSEWHERE

Radiotherapy given to relieve symptoms from cancer that has spread and cannot be cured is called *palliative radiotherapy*. Palliative radiotherapy may be given to almost any site of metastases. The treatment schedule will depend on the site of disease, the patient's state of health, and life expectancy. Most palliative treatment courses last from one day to two weeks.

Radiation therapy is only given to a specific part of the body. Most side effects are likely to be felt only in the area that is being treated. However, a patient receiving a program of chemotherapy combined with radiotherapy is likely to experience a combination of side effects from the two treatments. Some of these, such as diarrhea, may be more severe with the combined treatment than if the patient were receiving chemotherapy or radiation alone.

RADIATION CAUSES TWO MAIN SORTS OF SIDE EFFECTS

Radiation causes:

- ▶ Inflammation in the treated tissues that starts during the treatment and usually subsides within a few weeks of the completion of treatment. In fewer than 10% of patients, inflammation will persist and worsen with time, leading to intermittent bleeding from the rectum. This condition is called *radiation proctitis*.

▶ Damage to the small blood vessels in tissues that have received a high
dose of radiation. This is a gradually developing process that seems to
progress even after the radiotherapy course is long completed. It can
result in fragile tissue, scarring of the tissues that were radiated, and
some loss of normal function in the radiated tissues.

WHAT RADIOTHERAPY DOES NOT CAUSE

Radiotherapy treatments are painless, and, while some people experience
nausea, they do not usually vomit, or feel dizzy or lightheaded. Radiation
therapy does not cause hair loss unless the radiation is specifically directed
at the head or unless chemotherapy drugs being received cause hair to thin
or fall out. Except when brachytherapy is used (see Chapter 17), the patient
is *not* radioactive and therefore not a threat to friends, family, or pets. The
patient should feel well enough to drive back and forth to the clinic for radiotherapy treatments. Some patients even continue full-time employment during radiation treatment, although coping with chemotherapy at the same
time may make this difficult.

SIDE EFFECTS DURING TREATMENT

GENERAL SIDE EFFECTS

Tiredness

Although individuals vary widely in the extent to which they experience side
effects, the most common complaint is fatigue. About one person in three
will become noticeably tired. The cause of this is not known, but the best
remedy is to have an afternoon nap, maintain a balanced diet, and cut back
on stressful activities. After the radiation treatment is finished the fatigue
decreases gradually over the next few weeks to months. It is difficult to determine whether the fatigue is due to the treatments or to the psychological and
emotional stress that a diagnosis of cancer brings with it.

Emotional effects

Another effect of going to radiation therapy sessions is that it provides patients with a daily reminder of their cancer. This may cause feelings of anxiety or depression. Discussing these reactions with the radiation therapist and oncologist is important as patients will be assured that the feelings are normal and common. Asking questions or rearranging appointment times may help to maintain some control over the process. The emotional aspects of cancer are discussed in more detail in later chapters.

SIDE EFFECTS IN THE PELVIC AREA

The bowel

The usual pelvic radiation treatment includes most of the rectum. It may also affect some of the small intestine which could be lying in the pelvis. Radiotherapists try to avoid "hitting" the small intestine with radiotherapy but it does happen in some patients.

The small intestine is more sensitive to the effects of radiation than the rectum and produces the first symptoms, which are likely to be watery diarrhea with or without some stomach cramping. This starts about 10 to 14 days after the first treatment. With a short (one week) course of preoperative treatment, these symptoms are likely to appear just after surgery but, because of the effects of the surgery, probably won't be noticed. With a longer course of treatment either before or after surgery, diarrhea that may be made more severe by the effects of chemotherapy is likely. Most patients find that the diarrhea can be controlled by loperamide (brand name, Imodium). However, if the diarrhea doesn't respond to the doses recommended on the package, the oncologist should be informed as it is possible to become seriously dehydrated if the problem persists. Usually, diarrhea caused by inflammation of the small intestine subsides and becomes less of a problem within a week or so as the tissues are able to recover while treatment progresses.

Symptoms due to inflammation of the rectum (called *radiation proctitis*) develop three to four weeks into the course of treatment. As the inflammation builds, the rectum becomes more sensitive and the patient becomes less able to retain a large amount of stool or gas. Each day the patient is likely to have several small bowel movements. Some patients are already experiencing similar symptoms because of their cancer.

In contrast to inflammation of the small intestine, which produces loose or watery stools, inflammation of the rectum causes frequent small bowel movements which have a more normal consistency. However, the inflamed rectum often produces more mucus, which may be mixed with the stool or passed on its own. The symptoms of rectal inflammation can be reduced by the use of suppositories that contain anti-inflammatory medication such as hydrocortisone. The proctitis usually persists for a week or two after the radiotherapy has finished.

The bladder

The back of the bladder lies right in front of the rectum and will be within the radiation field. When the bladder becomes inflamed, symptoms such as more frequent urination and a burning sensation while urinating could develop. If this is severe, the oncologist should be informed as there is medication that can be helpful.

The prostate

The prostate gland lies in front of the rectum, just below the bladder. As such, it will usually lie within the radiation field and become inflamed. Some men, particularly those who already have some enlargement of the prostate, may experience increased difficulty urinating, although this is rarely a significant problem.

The vagina

The part of the vagina that is in the radiation field will become inflamed and may be uncomfortable. This will most likely limit sexual activity during and immediately after treatment. In the long term, there could be some vaginal dryness, which can be treated with lubricating creams or estrogen cream. Patients should seek their doctor's advice about which is the best to use in their individual case.

The skin

The skin at the anus and on the surrounding buttocks may be in the radiation field. In that case it will become inflamed and sore about three weeks after the treatment starts. The discomfort can be minimized by avoiding constipation, which is not usually a problem for those having chemotherapy as well as radiation. Also, the patient should avoid trauma such as vigorous wiping after a bowel movement or rubbing with a towel after a shower or bath. If the patient feels discomfort, the oncologist can recommend a cream to help reduce the inflammation. Skin should heal completely within two or three weeks after the completion of the radiotherapy.

Pelvic pain

Pelvic pain is a rare complication that is reported by about 5% of the patients who receive the short course preoperative treatment. Generally, it starts toward the end of the treatment course and usually responds well to painkillers such as acetaminophen (brand name, Tylenol) or ibuprofen (brand names, Advil or Motrin).

LATE RADIATION DAMAGE

Radiation can cause long-term damage to tissues. This damage is due to changes in small blood vessels that have been radiated. Fewer than 5% of patients are likely to develop significant symptoms from this complication. The most likely sites of this damage are in the small intestine and the rectum. Symptoms include intermittent abdominal cramping, diarrhea, and rectal bleeding that may be serious enough to cause anemia. Because these symptoms could be due to causes other than radiation damage, they should be reported by the patient to his or her doctor.

SEXUAL FUNCTION FOLLOWING PELVIC RADIOTHERAPY

When premenopausal women receive either the short or long course of pelvic radiotherapy, their ovaries become permanently damaged and they will enter menopause within two to three months. Having rectal cancer does not rule out the use of hormone replacement therapy. The decision about whether to use replacement therapy is one to be made with the family doctor after taking into account all the pros and cons. Postmenopausal women may experience vaginal discomfort or dryness that usually responds well to creams.

When it is necessary to treat the lower pelvis, radiation will permanently damage men's testes and they will become sterile. Occasionally, with cancers that are higher up in the rectum, there is the possibility of shielding the testes, although a risk of sterility from scattered radiation still exists.

Apart from this, the situation in men is somewhat less clear. There are to date no published reports about long term sexual function after treatment for rectal cancer with modern surgical and radiation techniques. There is no doubt that after surgery alone, a percentage of men will experience sexual problems such as the inability to get or maintain an erection, difficulty achieving an orgasm, or abnormal ejaculation. The proportion of patients experiencing these difficulties varies in different reports, from 13% to 40% depending on the patient's health before surgery and the type of surgery done. We know that radiotherapy alone given for prostate cancer results in sexual problems such as those mentioned above in between 30% and 40% of men who were sexually active before treatment. However, the radiation doses used to treat rectal cancer are significantly lower than those used for prostate cancer, and one would expect to see a lower incidence of complications with the lower rectal cancer doses. Overall, it is likely that surgery alone will lead to reduced sexual function in 15% to 20% of men and that the addition of radiotherapy either before or after the surgery will probably increase the risk to approximately 30%.

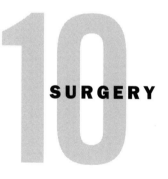

10

SURGERY

CHAPTER 20
THE DOCTOR HAS SUGGESTED SURGERY: WHAT SHOULD I DO?

A diagnosis of cancer will ultimately require action, but immediate treatment is rarely necessary. In most cases, the cancer will have been there for months or years, so whether you are treated today or a few weeks from now is not likely to make any difference. Taking some time to understand the disease, put things into perspective, and carefully assess your options for treatment is important. A cancer diagnosis strips you of your sense of control. Learning how to help yourself gives you back some of that control.

Today, patients with cancer interact with a team of health care providers as they move through the phases of diagnosis, staging, treatment, and recovery. You are part of the team and have a role to play—learning about the disease, hearing the options, discussing your needs with your family and friends, and coming to a comfortable decision about what you want.

Although long delays are not a good thing, you should not be rushed or pushed into accepting a treatment plan before you are ready, even if it means requesting a second opinion or waiting a little longer for surgery. You should feel informed and secure in the knowledge that the treatment you are about to undergo has been adequately explained and makes sense to you. Also, you should feel confident in the physicians and health care workers providing the treatment.

CHOOSING A SURGEON

How can you find the best surgeon for you? Usually, one surgeon cannot be singled out who is best for everyone in all circumstances. The ideal surgeon is knowledgeable about all aspects of your surgery and current practices, as well as being skillful in the operating room. Your surgeon should be someone with whom you feel confident. If you feel uncomfortable about requesting a second opinion or a different surgeon, you must push yourself to overcome that hesitation as it is essential that you feel confident in your medical care.

Most patients leave the choice of surgeon to their family doctor. This is fine provided you have confidence in both your family doctor and his or her choice. However, family practitioners may not be in a position to refer you to the best surgeon for your case because of standardized referral habits or because they work in a restrictive group practice. Also, remember that your doctor knows the surgeon as a colleague and not from a patient's perspective. If you have a good relationship with your doctor or have already discussed your cancer with an oncologist, you may simply need a surgeon who has good surgical technique.

Recommendations by friends tend to be based on the quality of the surgeon's bedside manner. Keep in mind that the best surgeons do not necessarily possess the warmest bedside manner. You should, however, be able to ask the surgeon questions and get satisfactory answers. Good information about surgeons can be obtained from local support and advocacy groups for colorectal cancer.

Many local cancer clinics have colorectal cancer policy groups. Surgeons participating in such a group will be aware of current trends and practices and may be more able to respond to your questions.

CHAPTER 21
CONVENTIONAL SURGERY FOR COLORECTAL CANCER

Operations for colorectal cancer are major ones. They are performed in the operating room of a hospital and require a general anesthetic. The operations may last anywhere from an hour-and-a-half to five hours depending on the degree of difficulty. Patients are positioned on their back, and may have their legs elevated in stirrups if the surgeon needs to insert instruments into the anus during the operation.

There are three principal ways of operating on colorectal cancer. The traditional way is to remove the cancer through an incision in the abdominal wall. Recently, some surgeons have begun removing colorectal cancer laparoscopically, a technique that involves the use of multiple long, narrow instruments passed through a group of tiny incisions in the abdominal wall. Finally, there is the rare situation in which a very small and superficial rectal cancer may be treated entirely through the anus (called *localized treatment*).

TRADITIONAL OPERATIONS

Traditional operations are, by far, the most common type of colorectal cancer operations. They involve an incision of 10 to 25 cm (4 to 10 inches) long in the abdominal wall, through which the surgeon removes the cancerous segment of bowel (Figure 18). Abdominal wall incisions for these procedures are usually vertically oriented, through the midline of the abdomen.

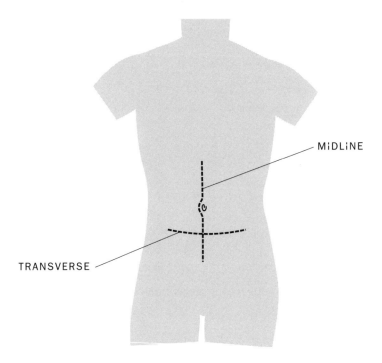

MiDLiNE

TRANSVERSE

Figure 18. *Incisions for traditional colorectal cancer operations.*

TRADITIONAL OPERATIONS FOR COLON CANCER

For the most part, operations for cancer of the colon are straightforward and consist of meticulous removal of the cancerous segment (called the *specimen*) and its accompanying lymph node tissues, followed by stapling together the ends of the remaining colon. The point where the two ends of the remaining bowel are joined is called the *anastomosis*.

Traditional operations balance the requirements for adequate removal of cancer and lymph nodes, and preservation of enough normal tissue. The choice of operation depends upon where the cancer lies. These traditional operations include the following (Figure 19):

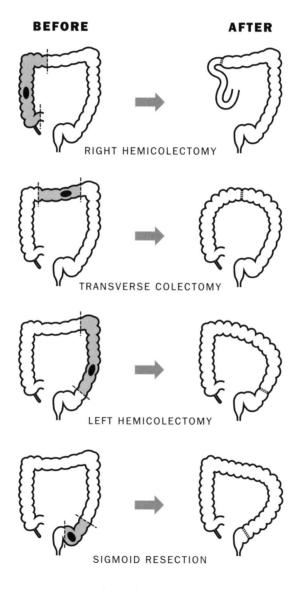

BEFORE　　　　　　　　　**AFTER**

RIGHT HEMICOLECTOMY

TRANSVERSE COLECTOMY

LEFT HEMICOLECTOMY

SIGMOID RESECTION

Figure 19. *Traditional operations for colon cancer.*

Right hemicolectomy

In a *right hemicolectomy*, cancer of the cecum or ascending colon is generally removed along with the entire ascending colon. An anastomosis is created between the end of the small intestine and the right side of the transverse colon.

Transverse colectomy

In a *transverse colectomy*, cancer in the transverse colon is removed with the entire transverse colon. The ascending colon is then anastomosed to the descending colon.

Left hemicolectomy

In a *left hemicolectomy*, cancer of the descending colon is removed with the entire descending colon, a portion of the left transverse colon, and the upper part of the sigmoid colon. The transverse colon is anastomosed to the upper sigmoid colon.

Sigmoid resection

In a *sigmoid resection*, cancer of the sigmoid colon requires removal of the sigmoid colon with anastomosis between the descending colon and rectum.

TRADITIONAL OPERATIONS FOR RECTAL CANCER

Surgery for rectal cancer is more difficult than surgery for colon cancer. Whereas a surgeon with modest surgical experience can achieve cure rates for colon cancer that are comparable to those from most leading centers in the world, the same surgeon would require much more training and experience to have this degree of success when dealing with rectal cancer.

The rectum lies deep within the bony pelvis, which may be so narrow that the surgeon has difficulty even passing a hand down to the cancer. This creates a situation where there may be a tendency for the less experienced surgeon to compromise on the adequacy of the removal of both the cancer (and a healthy margin of normal bowel on either side of it) and the adjacent lymph nodes. To accomplish a complete resection within the narrow confines of the pelvis requires a significant amount of skill and determination. In addition, there are large and fragile vessels in the pelvis that can bleed vigorously if torn, and tiny nerves that have an enormous impact on the patient's quality of life (sexual and bladder function) if they are damaged.

From the anus upward, the rectum is approximately 15 to 19 cm (10 to 12 inches) long. It is useful to consider it divided into thirds when deciding which operation is best (Figure 20). Cancers of the rectum lie in the upper, middle, or lower third. The upper third of the rectum is fairly easy to operate on as it is easily reached from within the abdomen. The middle third may be easy or difficult, and the lowest third is the hardest as it lies the deepest within the bony pelvis.

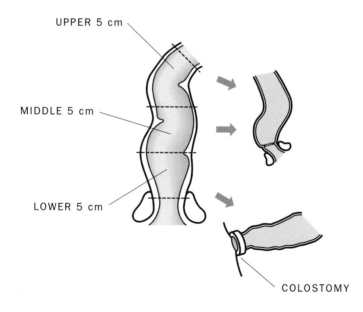

UPPER 5 cm

MIDDLE 5 cm

LOWER 5 cm

COLOSTOMY

Figure 20. *Rectal thirds. Upper third and middle third rectal cancers can usually be removed without colostomy. Lower third cancers often require colostomy.*

Anterior resection for rectal cancer

Any operation in which the cancerous portion of the rectum is removed and an anastomosis made (the remaining ends are joined) is called an *anterior resection* (Figure 21). This removes the cancer and adjacent lymph nodes while allowing the patient to continue having bowel movements through the anus.

Abdominoperineal resection for rectal cancer

An operation in which the cancerous portion of the rectum is removed along with the anus is called an *abdominoperineal resection* (Figure 21). Since there is nothing left to join the end of the colon to, it is sewn to an opening in the abdomen called a *colostomy*. Stool then empties from the colostomy into an *appliance* (colostomy bag) instead of coming out through the anus. The abdominoperineal operation is performed on low rectal cancers (usually lower third cancers) when it is felt that the anal sphincter must be sacrificed in order to ensure the greatest chance for cure. This is because the cancer is so low that it is lying extremely close to the anal sphincter, or has invaded it.

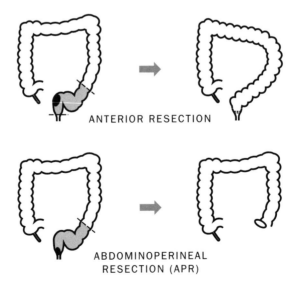

ANTERIOR RESECTION

ABDOMINOPERINEAL
RESECTION (APR)

Figure 21. *Anterior resection and abdominoperineal resection operations for rectal cancer.*

How low can anterior resection go?

Understandably, most patients would prefer to have an anterior resection with preservation of the anus rather than an abdominoperineal operation with a permanent colostomy. It is frequently possible to retain the anus even with a fairly low rectal cancer. However, it has not always been this way. As recently as the 1980s middle and lower third rectal cancers were thought not treatable by anterior resection since techniques did not permit anastomosis so low in the pelvis, and it was assumed that the cure rates would suffer if the all of the rectum and anus were not removed. Since then, advances in instrumentation and surgical technique, combined with a better understanding of these cancers, has led surgeons to treat most middle third rectal cancers by anterior resection, thus preserving the anus. The *EEA* (end-to-end anastomosis) staple gun (see below) makes low anastomoses possible.

As a general guideline, lower third rectal cancers can be felt by the examiner's finger inserted into the anus. This used to be an absolute sign that the anus had to be removed at surgery. Today, however, some lower third rectal cancers may be treated with anterior resection, provided there is no cancer in the surrounding sphincter muscles. When these operations are done by highly trained surgeons, leaving the anus in place should not compromise the cancer cure. Whether a lower third rectal cancer can be treated effectively by an anterior resection or whether the anus needs to be removed with the cancer depends on the physical examination, results of diagnostic tests, and the surgeon's experience and technical skill. Getting a second surgical opinion prior to undergoing surgery for a lower third rectal cancer can sometimes clarify which operation is best.

The choice of operation may have to wait until surgery is underway

Some low rectal cancers sit at a position where the surgeon isn't able to tell whether the anus can be saved until part of the dissection has been performed. If, after cutting away some of the attachments of the rectum, there is found to be enough normal rectum below the cancer for an anastomosis, the surgeon will proceed with an anterior resection. If, however, dissection fails to produce enough normal rectum below the cancer, an abdominoperineal resection must be done.

In situations where it is not certain which operation will be performed until surgery is underway, the patient should, as much as possible, be psychologically prepared for a colostomy. Also, the patient's abdomen should be marked ahead of time for a potential colostomy site in case it is required (See Chapter 43).

Total mesorectal excision—The new gold standard in rectal cancer surgery
Recently it has been found that careful management of the rectal lymph node tissues during surgery for rectal cancer (either anterior resection or abdominoperineal resection operations) greatly minimizes the chances of a rectal cancer recurring in the pelvis.

Lymphatic fluid draining from a rectal cancer flows initially to adjacent lymph nodes in the fatty tissue lying directly behind the rectum. Thus, there may be microscopic cancer cells in the lymph nodes of this area. This tissue, consisting of fat, lymphatic vessels, and lymph nodes, is called the *mesorectum* (see figures 8a and 8b in Chapter 2). The mesorectum is surrounded by a membrane called the *mesorectal fascia* that contains it and keeps it separate from adjacent pelvic tissues.

Surgeons now attempt to remove the entire mesorectum intact without damaging the mesorectal fascia. This is quite different from previous surgical techniques where surgeons would typically cut into the mesorectum. By removing the entire mesorectum package in one piece, the surgeon hopes to avoid spilling cancer cells or leaving cancerous lymph nodes behind. This new method of removing a rectal cancer is called *total mesorectal excision (TME)* and has greatly reduced the likelihood of rectal cancer recurring in the pelvis (Figure 22).

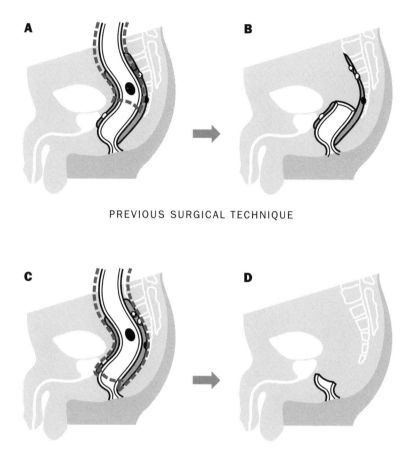

PREVIOUS SURGICAL TECHNIQUE

NEW (TME) TECHNIQUE

Figure 22. *The old and new forms of rectal cancer surgery. Images A and B show how rectal cancer used to be removed. The mesorectum with potentially malignant lymph nodes was left behind (B). Images C and D show complete removal of the mesorectum (total mesorectal excision) with the remaining short rectal stump ready for anastomosis (D).*

THE EEA (END-TO-END ANASTOMOSIS) STAPLER

The development of the end-to-end anastomosis stapler has been a tremendous advance in rectal cancer surgery. The stapler permits the surgeon to anastomose (join) two ends of bowel together deep in the pelvis. Before this stapler was developed, these very low anastomoses were sewn by hand, a procedure that is very difficult to do well, particularly in an individual with a low rectal cancer deep within the confines of a narrow pelvis. The stapler has made anastomoses possible whereas previously an abdominoperineal resection with a permanent colostomy might have been necessary.

Figure 23 illustrates how this stapler works. The two ends of the bowel are put inside the stapler. The stapler is closed and the instrument fires a circular double row of dozens of tiny staples through the bowel's ends. The many small staples make a more reliable anastomosis than can be done by hand.

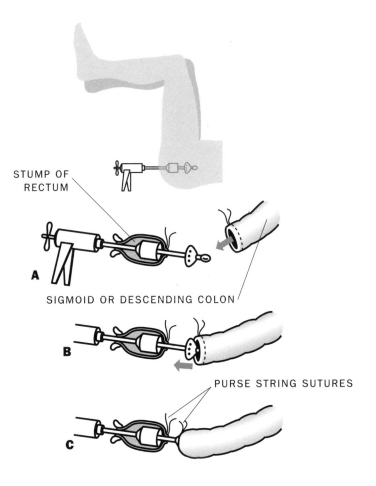

STUMP OF RECTUM

A

SIGMOID OR DESCENDING COLON

B

PURSE STRING SUTURES

C

Figure 23. *The EEA (end-to-end anastomosis) stapler.*

CHAPTER 22
PREPARING FOR AND RECOVERING FROM SURGERY

WAITING FOR ADMISSION TO HOSPITAL

In some hospitals, admission for surgery may be precisely booked ahead of time by the surgeon's office staff. The patient will be given a firm date and time to go to the hospital admission desk. In other hospitals, patients are placed on a waiting list for surgery and are contacted to go into hospital when a bed becomes available.

The waiting list system may provide very short notice to patients when a bed comes available, so it is important that the hospital is able to reach patients promptly and that the patient keep his or her schedule flexible pending admission. It is not uncommon for a call to be put out as late as the evening before surgery. If you do not have a personal cell phone, this is a good time to get one. Give the number to your surgeon's office and the hospital admitting department and keep the phone with you at all times throughout your treatment and recovery so you will not have to worry about missing important calls such as these. Be careful not to disclose the phone number to anyone other than those required to know it or those very close to you. You want only important calls on this phone until you have recovered.

If you are in Canada, you need to be aware that treatment scheduling is sometimes complicated by lack of ready resources. You must be prepared for some delays. It is not unheard of for a patient to be called in for surgery and undergo admission to hospital, only to be sent home to wait again because the operating room did not come available as planned.

WHAT YOU CAN DO TO PREPARE

There may be some things you can do while waiting for admission that will improve your chances of having a smooth operation and recovery. If you reduce or quit smoking you may lessen your chances of postoperative chest complications such as pneumonia. If you have significant dental problems such as untreated tooth decay, get that dealt with before surgery since areas of infection or tooth decay can increase the chances of postoperative chest complications.

Heavy alcohol consumption prior to surgery can also lead to postoperative problems. These can vary from mild jitteriness to life-threatening delirium tremens (DTs). If you consume substantial amounts of alcohol regularly, reduce your alcohol intake promptly and let your surgeon know about it. He or she may choose to delay surgery for a short period to help you prepare and may recruit the assistance of a specialist in this area who can be standing by postoperatively if needed.

If you have diabetes, high blood pressure, heart disease, or any other significant medical problem, the preoperative period is an excellent time to seek urgent review of these systems by your specialist. The specialist can optimize the management of each system prior to surgery and can plan to work with your surgeon in the postoperative phase if necessary.

YOU'RE IN!

WELCOME TO CHAOS?

A number of admission procedures will be required, so come prepared with all the patience you can muster. A variety of people will ask you a lot of questions, some you will have already answered many times over. There may be delays, foul-ups, snarky personnel and people who seem totally unconcerned with the seriousness of your problem. Most disturbing of all is that growing feeling that everyone working in the place is totally incompetent. What to do when this happens? Relax.

The force and energy of the hospital's critical services and personnel will be mustered for you when you need it (but often not before, or after). Hospitals are big places where all kinds of life events take place, particularly in major centers where emergencies are frequent. The priorities of physicians, nurses, orderlies, and admitting clerks may be suddenly altered, leaving you in a frustrating holding pattern. If you conclude that the place is in total chaos, you will not be the first to have done so. However, this observation is far from the truth.

The best way to get through the preoperative period in hospital (and much of the stay following surgery) is to just grin and bear it. Your lifeline is your confidence in your surgeon and the knowledge that in all this apparent chaos, there is order, and the hospital will provide the right treatment at the right time. While you may be sitting in the lurch wondering why you have been suddenly deserted, there is likely a very ill person down the hall who requires the immediate attention of the eight highly qualified people at his or her bedside. This is what hospitals are all about.

HOSPITAL ADMISSION

Your first meeting will be with the admissions clerk. Identification and basic personal information is recorded. Financial or insurance information will be requested, so make sure you bring identification and health care cards with you. From the admissions desk you will be directed or escorted to your hospital room.

NURSING ADMISSION

Once you are on the ward, a nurse carries out a nursing admission. The nurse will record basic information regarding your health and current problem, then give you a brief examination that includes a measurement of your weight and assessment of your vital signs (heart rate, breathing rate, blood pressure, and temperature.)

DOCTOR ADMISSION

In a non-university hospital, a copy of the consultation note from the surgeon's office will have been sent to the hospital and this will serve as the source of medical information regarding the problem and any physical examinations. The surgeon may be required to update that information after you arrive.

In a university hospital, a medical admission is done by the medical student, intern, or surgical resident (both interns and residents are physicians completing their training). You will be asked to relate your medical history to this person yet again. A list of the tests already completed will be recorded, along with the responses to a variety of basic medical questions. Then the examiner will do a physical examination. Depending upon the organization of the particular teaching program at the hospital, the residents may later arrive as a group to see you, often with the chief resident. The chief resident is responsible for ensuring that an appropriate medical admission and interpretation of questions and findings are made, along with organizing last minute tests and preparations for surgery.

SURGICAL RESIDENTS

Many hospitals are affiliated with universities and have a responsibility to teach surgical residents. While patients usually accept that their busy surgeons require the assistance of the residents on the ward, they may become anxious when they learn that the residents might be participating in and, in some cases, performing their operation.

Some patients insist that the residents not even be allowed into the operating room in order to ensure that only their surgeon does the operation. If surgeons complied with such requests, not only would they be in jeopardy of losing their university appointment, they would definitely be reducing the patient's chances of getting through the operation without a complication. The fact is that most major operations are difficult and dangerous when performed by a single surgeon, and the presence of the resident may be critical to the success of the procedure. A major operation is a team effort in which residents and other assistants play an important role.

From the point of view of the person who does the operation, the to-and-fro of steps required between operator and assistant is in some cases so evenly spread that one would be hard-pressed to say who did more work, the surgeon or the first assistant. In some cases, the senior resident may actually be a better operator because residents frequently operate around the clock and have done so for three to eight years. By the time they are nearing the end of their training, some are very skilled indeed.

A more important question than "Who does the operation?" is "Who is directing the operation?" With the surgeon present at the operating table assisting and guiding the resident, the result will be as good as or better than if the surgeon had done it solo. This is the basis of a strong surgical training program and excellent patient care. The presence of the senior surgeon insures that mature surgical judgment prevails at important points of decision, while his or her critical eye makes careful note that all technical steps are completed accurately.

There is no need to feel any less confident when some of your care is administered by a resident and that he or she may participate in your operation. It is your right, however, to expect close supervision of residents by the staff surgeon in the operating room, and frequent consultation by the residents with the senior surgeon when difficult decisions must be made on the ward.

PREPARING FOR SURGERY

BLOOD CROSS-MATCH

In most cases, blood will be "cross-matched" for your surgery. This means that a sample of your blood will be tested and compatible blood found and reserved for you in case a blood transfusion is required during your operation. Your need for blood will depend upon the degree of difficulty of the operation and your starting blood level (hemoglobin level).

Colon cancer surgery differs from rectal cancer surgery in the requirement for blood transfusion. In most cases of colon cancer surgery, a blood transfusion is not required. Rectal cancer surgery is generally more difficult and the blood loss higher, making the requirement for blood transfusion more likely.

In the old days, surgeons used to give blood to patients who had a slightly low blood count before or after surgery. Today, as a result of the small but real hazards associated with blood transfusions, along with the expense and difficulty of obtaining blood, physicians and surgeons have modified their use of blood and blood products dramatically and now give blood only when it is absolutely necessary.

As a result of the AIDS crisis, programs have been developed in which patients can bank their own blood before an operation so that if blood is required, they receive their own blood back. This is called *autologous* blood donation. The timing for this can be tricky for cancer patients since enough time between the donation and surgery must pass to allow the patients to build up their blood level again for the operation. Since cancer surgery is usually done within a few weeks of diagnosis, there may not be enough time. To find out whether there is a personal blood banking system in your area and whether you are a suitable candidate, speak to your surgeon and the local Red Cross or hospital blood bank.

You have the right to refuse blood if you wish. If that is your choice, you should ensure that your surgeon and other medical personnel are clearly notified of this. In order to protect the doctor and hospital, you may be required to sign a release to this effect.

BOWEL PREPARATION

Before surgery, it is important that the bowel be cleansed of feces. Feces consist primarily of bacteria, so any spillage during surgery can result in an infection. In order to cleanse the colon before surgery, patients are given a *bowel preparation (bowel prep)*. The bowel may be prepped either by drinking large volumes (four liters; 16 cups) of a specially prepared salty fluid, or by taking lesser volumes of a magnesium-based purgative. Bowel preparation may be done in the hospital the night before surgery or by the patient at home just prior to admission to hospital. More detail on bowel preparation is provided in the Appendix.

ANTIBIOTIC COVERAGE

Antibiotics given just before colorectal operations and continued for a brief period following surgery have been found to decrease infection rates. Some surgeons prescribe oral tablets for this purpose; others order intravenous antibiotics to be started just before the operation. If you are allergic to any antibiotics, be sure to remind your surgeon or the residents when the antibiotics are ordered.

MARKING THE SITE FOR A POSSIBLE ABDOMINAL STOMA

A *stoma* is an opening on the abdomen that an end of the intestine is brought through. The feces then empty into an *appliance* (bag) that is taped to the skin around the stoma. A stoma may be permanent or temporary. Chapter 43 is dedicated to a discussion on stomas. A stoma is sometimes required as part of a colorectal cancer operation. If there is a possibility that a stoma may be needed in your case, the surgeon should discuss this with you.

If a stoma is necessary or even if it is just a possibility, the abdomen should be assessed before the operation to determine the best site for the opening. A *stoma therapist* or *enterostomal therapist* is a nurse who specializes in finding the right place for stomas and assisting you with your stoma and appliances following surgery. The stoma therapist has experience in knowing which stoma position will be most comfortable and easiest to manage on your abdomen. The placement should take account of the individual attributes of your abdomen, such as the hills and valleys, wrinkles and scars, and so on. The enterostomal therapist may ask to see how you wear your pants to assess the level of the beltline (something that should be avoided) and may ask you to bend over to see how the skin on your abdominal wall moves during activity. Combining all of this information, the stoma therapist will choose a preferred location and will mark it with an indelible marker so that the surgeon can identify it during the operation if required. It is important that this is done beforehand as the operating table is not the ideal place to select a stoma site.

Preoperative marking of the preferred stoma site is often overlooked on a busy hospital surgery ward. If you have been told that you may require a stoma, you must be proactive in ensuring that the stoma therapist comes by before your operation. Remind your nurse to contact the stoma therapist on your arrival to the ward.

ABDOMINAL SHAVE

Removal of all hair on the abdomen used to be a routine measure before an operation. Recently, however, there has been some evidence to suggest that shaving, unless done just before surgery, may lead to an increase in the wound infection rate by creating small cuts in which bacteria may grow. For this reason, abdominal shaving is not nearly as common as it used to be and is a matter of the surgeon's preference. The evidence that it is harmful is not very strong, so you should leave this decision up to your surgeon.

A VISIT BY THE ANESTHETIST

At some point before your operation, you will meet an anesthetist. He or she will review your medical history and ask you about prior anesthetic experiences. You are entitled to enquire about the various means of anesthesia that might be suitable for your operation, and express your preference. For most colorectal operations, a general anesthetic is required, meaning that you will be unconscious during the operation. Occasionally, a pure spinal anesthetic may be possible, but this is usually reserved for the elderly. If a spinal anesthetic is used for colorectal patients, it is often in combination with a general anesthetic —the addition of the spinal anesthetic to the general anesthetic sometimes results in a reduction in postoperative pain. Your anesthetist should be able to present the various choices and recommend what is best for you.

ON THE WAY TO THE OPERATING ROOM

An hour or two before your scheduled operation, you will be greeted by an orderly or porter who will transport you to the surgery floor, usually by stretcher. You will not go directly to the operating room but will more likely be taken to a holding area where your identification will be checked and a nurse will make sure you understand what you are there for and that you have signed a consent form for surgery. When the patient scheduled before you has left the operating room, the room has been thoroughly cleaned and the anesthetist has replenished his or her supplies, you will be wheeled into the operating room. Since one can never predict exactly how long each case will take, you should not expect your operation to start exactly at the time it is scheduled unless you are the first case of the day. In most busy hospitals, if you arrive in the operating room anywhere within a couple of hours of the posted schedule, you are doing just fine. Expect such delays so they won't upset you; it is all part of life in a hospital.

Once you are in the operating room, the anesthetist and nurses will check that they have the right person for the right surgeon and the right operation. You will be moved onto what is usually a very narrow and firm operating table and an intravenous drip will be started in your arm, unless you already have one. You will note a lot of activity in the room, and unfamiliar equipment and sounds as nurses and doctors make preparations for your procedure. You may or may not have a chance to talk to your surgeon before you are anesthetized. Sometimes the surgeon is finishing another case or coming up from the ward when the anesthetist puts you to sleep in order to keep on schedule. Most anesthetists will not put you to sleep unless they know the surgeon is down the hall. If you wish, you may request that you not be anesthetized until you have had a chance to see the surgeon in the operating room.

IMMEDIATELY POST-OP

BREATHING ASSISTANCE

During a general anesthetic, both sleeping (anesthetic) and paralyzing drugs (muscle relaxants) are given. The former produces unawareness during surgery and the latter relax the muscles so the surgeon can get at the area to be operated on. Newer drugs may combine both effects in one. During general anesthesia, patients are so deeply asleep and without muscle control that breathing must be done for them. To facilitate this, the anesthetist slides a

small (endotracheal) tube through the mouth and into the windpipe shortly
after the patient reaches unconsciousness (Figure 24). The tube is connected
to a ventilator that moves air in and out of the lungs during the operation.
The anesthetist carefully monitors the ventilator's performance during the
operation and is ready to intervene at any moment if problems develop.

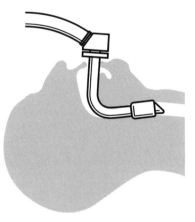

Figure 24. *Endotracheal tube.*

As the surgeons sew the wound closed, the anesthetist begins to reduce
the concentration of anesthetic gas or intravenous anesthetic medications or
gradually reverses the anesthetic medications with specific antidotes. While
the bandages are applied, you will start to drift toward consciousness and
begin trying to breathe on you own. When you are awake enough to breathe
safely without the ventilator's assistance, the anesthetist will remove the
endotracheal tube from your throat while talking reassuringly to reorient
you to the unfamiliar operating room surroundings. Orderlies, doctors, and
nursing staff move you from the operating table onto a stretcher that will
carry you down the hall to the recovery room.

NOTIFYING YOUR SIGNIFICANT OTHER

In most cases, there is someone you will want the surgeon to contact when your operation is over. It is important that this person's name and phone number be clearly written on the chart and that the person is standing by awaiting the call. While you are being wheeled to the recovery room, your surgeon is reaching for the phone to contact this person. The surgeon will describe what he or she has found (if this is your wish), what was done, and how the operation went. On the rarest of occasions, if there is a difficult decision to make during an operation, the surgeon may want to contact this person while you are still anesthetized to consult with him or her. Make sure that there is only one person to call. The surgeon will not have time to involve a variety of people at this point. It should be clear that this "patient representative" will act as the sole liaison between family, friends, and the surgeon until you are once again able to assume the role.

THE RECOVERY ROOM

The anesthetist goes with the patient to the recovery room and stays close by until he or she is certain that there are no problems. The surgeon provides the recovery room nurses with a list of orders that cover a variety of areas, including directions for pain relief, timing of appropriate blood tests, and instructions for giving antibiotics or other medications.

Most patients can't remember much about their stay in the recovery room, although they may respond appropriately (but slowly) to questions and commands while they are there. Mostly, they sleep, groan, or smile bravely after being reassured that their operation is over and that they have survived.

The amount of time spent in the recovery room varies with the type of operation as well as with hospital policy. In general, the patient stays in the recovery area until he or she no longer needs the one-to-one attention. Some patients remain in the recovery room overnight or longer, if further observation or treatment is warranted. Many hospitals have a policy requiring that patients be transferred to the intensive care unit should things still not be going well after an overnight stay in the recovery room.

Beyond ensuring that patients are as comfortable as possible, recovery room nurses fulfill two critical roles: they make sure that the anesthetic has been appropriately reversed, and they watch for surgical complications.

INADEQUATE REVERSAL

Reversing is a term used to describe the procedure involved in waking a patient after anesthetic. It may be done simply by turning off anesthetic agents (inhaled gases) or by giving intravenous reversing agents. Sometimes a combination of methods is used. Occasionally, a patient who appeared to be waking up adequately drifts back into an anesthetic state in the recovery room and is in danger of suffocation from underbreathing. Recovery room nurses are on the lookout for this problem and when they notice it, the patient will be roused by talking, physical stimulation (like pinching) or by certain drugs that wake the patient up.

BLEEDING

Bleeding in the recovery room does not happen often, but when it does, it can be very serious and must be identified quickly. Bleeding at this stage usually means that a tie on a blood vessel has come away, or that a divided blood vessel that was not bleeding during the operation now is.

Identifying postoperative bleeding requires skill and experience because it is rarely visible. The bleeding is usually inside, at the site of surgery, and can only be recognized by watching the patient's vital signs (pulse, blood pressure, respiratory rate) and abdomen.

In some operations, the surgeon will leave a *drain* (plastic tube) in the wound so that normal amounts of fluid and blood may be evacuated. One end of the drain is placed in the operative area and the other end is brought out through the skin and connected to a gentle suction pump. An excessive amount of blood coming through the drain is one of the easier ways to identify abnormal postoperative bleeding. This is one of the reasons why some surgeons use drains.

If the nurse identifies signs of bleeding, the surgeon will be called promptly to examine the patient in the recovery room. The surgeon may decide to take the patient back to the operating room and re-anesthetize him or her. The abdomen or other operative site will be reopened, the accumulated blood evacuated and the bleeding points tied off.

BACK ON THE WARD

Most patients recovering from colon or rectal surgery will spend five to 10 days on the ward. When departure time finally rolls around, they are usually quite pleased to be saying farewell.

PAIN

Pain after surgery is unavoidable. Fortunately, much of it can be controlled with strong pain killers available in hospital. The most common regimen for managing surgical pain in the first few postoperative days is buttock injections of either morphine or Demerol every three to four hours. Don't fear that you will turn into a drug addict or feel guilty about needing the injections. After all, this is precisely why medical science developed these medications! As the third or fourth day after surgery passes, the need for these strong drugs diminishes. Once eating is resumed, oral (tablet) pain killers are usually adequate.

THE INTRAVENOUS

Prior to your surgery, an intravenous line will be inserted into a vein in your hand or arm. The fluid infused through the line is a salt solution that closely matches the salt concentrations in your blood. The intravenous provides you with the fluid you would normally be drinking, in order to keep up with your body's fluid losses. The rate of infusion is adjusted according to how much fluid and blood you lost at surgery and what the estimated ongoing loss is after surgery. The intravenous line generally stays in place until you can drink adequate amounts of fluid yourself. An advantage to having an intravenous line is that medications can be given through the line in some cases, avoiding the need for further injections.

URINE OUTPUT

Urine volume is an important piece of postoperative information. The volume of a patient's urine reflects the amount of fluid and blood in the circulatory system. After major surgery, fluid weeps into the irritated tissues of the abdominal cavity and the level of fluid in the veins and arteries can drop. This is known as *third space loss*. When third space losses are great, the kidneys try to retain fluid by reducing urine output. This is fine, up to a point. However, if the circulating blood volume gets too low, the kidneys and other organs become starved of fluid and begin to suffer irreparable damage. By keeping track of the amount of a patient's urine, third space losses can be estimated. If the urine output is too low, more intravenous fluid will be given to compensate.

In order to carefully monitor urine output in postoperative patients (for whom getting up and going to the bathroom frequently would be too burdensome), a urinary catheter is used. This is a tube inserted into the bladder through the urethra. When the catheter is in place, urine flows freely from the bladder into a bag hanging on the bedrails. Because the patient is unable to stop the flow of urine through the catheter, an hourly urine output can be measured.

Third space losses become insignificant after three to four days following surgery, and at that time, the urinary catheter is removed.

DIET (OR LACK OF IT)

The intestine is very sensitive to manipulation by the surgeon. It reacts to the insult of being picked up and pushed around by going into a kind of shock called an *ileus*. For a period of three to seven days postoperatively, the normal contractions in the intestine cease, and the bowel becomes filled with tissue fluids and swallowed air. If you were to eat during this period, you would become bloated and vomit. Sometimes, even without eating, vomiting and bloating will occur during the ileus phase following surgery. To prevent this, a *nasogastric tube* may be inserted through the nose and passed down the esophagus into the stomach during surgery. Its purpose is to continuously suck out fluid and swallowed air. The tube is normally left in place until the ileus resolves, three to seven days following surgery.

The most reliable sign that the intestine is once again functioning normally is the passage of gas. Nowhere in life is passing wind more significant than on the surgery ward after intestinal surgery. Everything is on hold until that moment. The arrival of gas means that the intestine is once again ready for food. It also reassures the surgeon that the patient has passed through the most critical part of the recovery period because anastomotic leak, one of the most dreaded of postoperative complications, rarely occurs once the patient has begun to pass gas.

Before passing gas, your diet is non-existent, particularly, if there is a nasogastric tube in place. You cannot be fed food or fluid as this would just come up the tube or block it. While the nasogastric tube is in place, you will be given only intravenous fluid. There is a bit of glucose in intravenous fluid, but its nutritional value is minimal and, for the most part, this is a period of controlled starvation.

Once the ileus has passed, diet is reinstated. Initially, just sips of clear fluids may be given. Increased amounts of clear fluids are permitted the next day and full fluids such as soups are given on the day following that. Then, a normal diet is resumed.

YOUR ROLE IN THE POSTOPERATIVE PERIOD

Dismiss the idea that your postoperative period will be peaceful, and that you will lie in bed attended like a queen bee in a hive. Instead, you may find that your nurses unceremoniously kick you out of bed and force you to walk up and down the halls, even though walking causes you severe pain. They know that there are fewer surgical complications when patients are mobilized as soon as possible after surgery. In particular, there is less chance of developing blood clots in your legs, and intestinal function is thought to return more promptly in patients who get up and move about.

Deep breathing exercises are also important; there is a natural tendency to take shallow breaths following abdominal surgery because deep breaths hurt. Shallow breathing can lead to areas of collapse in the lungs, which may cause fever and lay the foundation for pneumonia. For this reason, patients are asked to force themselves to take three consecutive painfully deep breaths every 15 minutes when they are awake for at least the first week following abdominal surgery. These exercises should only be done lying flat in the bed as deep breaths in the sitting or standing position may result in faintness.

In many hospitals, physiotherapists assist with these important breathing exercises. Small plastic bedside devices called *incentive inspirometers* are available to allow the patient to measure his or her deep breathing efforts.

SHORT-TERM POSTOPERATIVE PSYCHOLOGICAL CHANGES

It is not uncommon for some reversible psychological changes to take place for a short time after major surgery. Sometimes called *postoperative confusion*, this occurs most often in patients over the age of 50 and is probably caused by a combination of the stress of surgery, unfamiliar surroundings, pain, anxiety, medications, separation from family, and a disrupted sleep cycle. The symptoms of postoperative confusion include anything from mild disorientation to real hallucinations. Previously placid individuals have been known to become anxious and aggressive. This can be frightening for both the patient and family.

Fortunately, postoperative confusion is temporary. Treatment may include a change of rooms, altered medication and, occasionally, a brief period of treatment by the psychiatric service. Serious infection and other medical problems can contribute to postoperative confusion, so it is important that they be ruled out. Provided there is no underlying problem, time may be the most important aspect of treatment. Sooner or later, if the person is otherwise doing well, he or she will come out of it and may or may not recall this difficult period. Those who do are often quite sorry about how they behaved and need to be reminded of how normal postoperative confusion is.

This simple type of confusion must be differentiated from the disturbance seen in patients who were excessive drinkers before surgery and who develop confusion and other symptoms of alcohol withdrawal during the postoperative period. Such patients may go on to develop delirium tremens (DTs), which, unlike simple postoperative confusion, may have serious medical implications.

STITCHES

Nowadays, the skin part of a wound may be closed with stitches, staples, or adhesive tape strips. Stitches and staples in the skin must be removed from three to 10 days after the operation. In general, stitches or staples left in the skin for more than seven days serve little purpose and are more likely to leave a visible stitch scar. Stitches under the skin, in the deeper tissues, are typically dissolvable over a period of several weeks, although some surgeons prefer non-dissolvable nylon material for these deeper tissues. Regardless of the surgeon's choice, the deep stitches are not designed to be removed.

METAL STAPLES

Many surgeons now use metal staplers to join the ends of the bowel together or to tie off blood vessels during surgery. They are generally made of titanium. While these staples do not dissolve and may be visible on an X-ray, you need not worry that they will set off alarms at airports.

A NOTE ABOUT VISITORS

Other than winning a lottery, there is little that can compete with a stay in the hospital for bringing friends and relatives out of the woodwork. Depending upon your personality and your medical condition following surgery, this may or may not please you. If it does not, the simplest way of avoiding the stress of attending to visitors is by not announcing to anyone other than your immediate family that you are going in for surgery. We sometimes advise patients to be "away on a vacation." For those individuals who manage to find out your secret, a "no visitors policy" (you can say that the surgeon insisted) will be strictly enforced if an order is written in the chart. This can be modified to permit special visitors.

GOING HOME

A DEPARTURE CHECKLIST

You are bound to have questions about your home rehabilitation and follow-up, so write them down and be prepared to go through the list when you see your doctor for the last time in hospital. The moment of discharge always feels like a small victory for any surgeon, and most are glad to take a few moments to answer some questions. By keeping a list, you are less likely to leave out an important concern.

Make sure you understand any instructions about temporary limitations of physical activity, discharge medications (ask that the appropriate prescriptions be left for you at the nursing station), dressing changes (if any), and follow-up. You may wish to leave something for the nursing staff, but this is totally voluntary. It is not appropriate to tip. Rather, a box of chocolates or nuts left at the nursing station for the ward staff is always appreciated.

THE FIRST THREE MONTHS

The first 12 weeks at home after major surgery are a time of major adjustment. Most people experience both physical and emotional challenges. This is a time of adjustment to the trauma of the surgery and the tasks of reintegration into family and work life. Physical problems will probably include intermittent bouts of abdominal pain, constipation, diarrhea, and fatigue, all of which should fade as the six to 12 week mark approaches. Constipation and diarrhea may both be treated effectively by fiber supplements such as Metamucil. Mood swings are common and feeling blue and crying are not unusual after such a challenging major life event.

The timing for returning to work depends upon the smoothness of the recovery period and the nature of your occupation. To permit the wound to regain its maximum strength, lifting more than two to four kg (five to 10 lbs.), the weight of a telephone book, or straining for the first three months, must be avoided. The person who works at a desk job can expect to return to work within six weeks of discharge from the hospital. Someone employed in a position requiring stressful physical work will require more time away, or a modification of the job until he or she is able to begin lifting again. Another factor to be taken into account is the potential requirement for postoperative chemotherapy and radiotherapy. These treatments may be time-consuming and will create their own recovery periods, and sometimes it is best to stay away from work until they have been concluded. Your physician is in the best position to help you weigh these various influences, plan with you an appropriate return, and provide the required documentation to your employers to ensure that your rights are protected.

HOW LONG DOES IT TAKE TO RECOVER FROM

MAJOR ABDOMINAL SURGERY?

Fatigue is the most long-lasting of the common postoperative symptoms. While other postoperative problems resolve within the first three to four months, it can take up to a year for a patient to fully recover his or her former energy level and stamina after colorectal surgery through the abdomen. Failure to understand this can lead to depression among those who are normally used to being very active. You must be gentle and patient with yourself, and with time, your energy will return.

CHAPTER 23
SURGICAL COMPLICATIONS

COMPLICATIONS ARE A FACT OF LIFE IN SURGERY

Complications are problems that can arise during or after an operation. They are more common than one might think, and they vary in significance from minor infections of the surgical wound to far more serious events.

The average person naturally assumes that complications do not arise in the practice of a well-trained, competent surgeon. Unfortunately, however, complications are a fact of life in surgery. If a surgeon does enough operations, eventually some of his or her patients will have complications. Surgeons of the highest quality do not deny their past complications but embrace them as important lessons in a career-long pursuit of the perfection they strive toward.

In major abdominal surgery, a surgeon who performs the identical careful operation on 100 patients will typically end up with 75 who sail through, 15 who have minor complications, seven who develop more serious complications, and up to three patients who experience life-threatening problems.

WHY DO COMPLICATIONS HAPPEN?

There are many reasons complications arise. They include factors related to the surgeon's judgment and technical skill, the type of operation performed, and the patient's underlying medical condition and ability to tolerate the operation.

SURGEON-RELATED FACTORS

Complication rates vary from surgeon to surgeon. Surgeons bring two elements to the treatment of their patients—technical skill and judgment. In some cases, the differences in complication rates are partly due to technical competence as some surgeons are better technicians than others. Technical skill related to a particular operation improves greatly when a surgeon performs that operation frequently, and most patients are best served by a surgeon that does their operation at least two or three times per month. But great technique alone is not enough. It is superior judgment that more often keeps patients safe. Surgical judgment influences the surgeon's choice of operation and timing of surgery, the myriad decisions made during an operation, and the best management of the patient postoperatively.

OPERATION-RELATED FACTORS

Some operations are harder to perform than others or are associated with a greater amount of trauma to the patient, so they would be expected to yield more frequent complications.

PATIENT-RELATED FACTORS

A surgeon who performs operations on very sick patients will almost certainly have a higher complication rate than one who operates on less sick patients, by virtue of the fact that ill patients are less able to tolerate the surgery. Patients who smoke, are diabetic, hypertensive, obese, and so on, all present increased risks for surgery. In addition, emergency operations are always accompanied by a higher complication rate than are elective, non-emergency procedures because emergency patients are, by definition, already in trouble. They are generally more ill than non-emergency patients, and there is less time to prepare them physically for the stress of surgery.

THE COMPLICATIONS

Complications may be classified as being intraoperative (during the operation), early postoperative (within 30 days following the operation) or late postoperative (more than 30 days following the operation). In addition, complications may be either directly or indirectly related to the operation. If a patient loses his or her sight after an eye operation, that is a complication directly related to the operation. If the patient were to develop an allergic reaction to the anesthetic used during the operation, that would be an indirect complication, as it had nothing to do with the type of operation itself, but was only the result of the patient having undergone surgery.

INTRAOPERATIVE COMPLICATIONS

There are a number of indirect complications that can occur during any operation. These include complications related to insertion of the intravenous catheters, breathing tubes, and other devices that are used to manage and monitor the anesthetized patient. Other indirect complications include stressed joints from awkward positioning on the operating table, or possible allergic (or other) reactions to medications used for anesthesia.

Intraoperative complications that are directly related to the operation usually consist of injuries to organs adjacent to the operating area.

Examples include:

- ► An injury to the spleen when attempting to remove a cancer of the transverse colon.
- ► An injury to the pelvic nerves controlling the bladder and ejaculation during dissection to remove a rectal cancer.

> ► An injury to the ureter when removing a cancer of the sigmoid colon. The ureter (the tube that takes urine from the kidney to the bladder) lies behind the sigmoid colon.

Careful surgeons are keenly aware of the proximity to the colon of these important structures, and such injuries should be uncommon in experienced hands.

EARLY POSTOPERATIVE COMPLICATIONS

In the early postoperative period, the most common indirect complications include fever, pneumonia, blood clots, transient psychological changes, and heart problems. Early postoperative direct complications are primarily related to leakage from the anastomosis (where the intestine is joined together after a segment has been removed).

Fever

Postoperative fever is very common. It is most often caused by small areas of collapse of a portion of the air spaces in the lungs, called *atelectasis*. This is usually the result of a combination of the effect of the inhaled anesthetic gas on lung membranes and the tendency for patients to take shallow breaths in the postoperative period because it hurts to take deep breaths. Fever from atelectasis usually occurs within 24 to 48 hours after surgery. Atelectasis is treated by postoperative chest physiotherapy that emphasizes deep-breathing exercises.

Pneumonia

Atelectasis may progress to *pneumonia* (infection of the lungs) if the airspaces are not opened promptly. Smokers and patients with emphysema or chronic bronchitis are at increased risk of postoperative pneumonia.

Wound infection

Infection of the surgical wound is fairly common. Infections typically occur three to four days following surgery and can be the cause of a delayed postoperative fever. An infected wound is treated by opening it to permit pus to drain. If the patient had a fever, the fever usually drops rapidly after this. If the wound is opened properly, antibiotics are rarely needed unless there is significant infection within the surrounding tissues, which is uncommon, or if the patient has an abnormal immune system or significant diabetes.

Blood clots

The human body responds to stress by increasing the clotting ability of the blood. Add to this the fact that patients don't move much because of their surgical pain, and one can understand the heightened risk for blood clots in the vessels of the legs and pelvis postoperatively. More significantly, these clots may travel up the veins and into the lungs, where they are called *pulmonary emboli*. Clots in the lungs lead to impaired lung function and can be very serious. Patients are encouraged to get out of bed and begin walking as soon as possible after surgery and are sometimes given platelet-inhibiting medications to prevent postoperative blood clots. If you have a history of previous blood clots, be sure to bring this to your surgeon's attention so that appropriate preventative measures can be provided.

Postoperative psychological changes

Temporary psychological changes are common during the postoperative period, and are frequently seen in elderly patients who have undergone major surgery. These changes may vary from mild to severe disorientation and personality change, and even transient psychosis. While these can be very disturbing for family members, they are almost always brief and can be managed with gentle and understanding nursing care. Occasionally, psychiatric assistance and a short course of medications may be required. Prolonged postoperative psychological change in an elderly patient may indicate that a stroke has occurred and appropriate investigations need to be made.

Heart attack

Patients with disease in the arteries that supply blood to the heart (called the *coronary* arteries) are at risk for heart attack during or following stressful surgery. Current methods of preoperative evaluation and anesthetic management during surgery have greatly reduced the rates of this complication, but it does still occur in some cases. An updated cardiology consultation preoperatively is a prudent measure if you have heart disease.

Anastomotic leak

In colorectal surgery, the most serious early direct complication is leakage from the anastomosis, where the bowel is sewn or stapled together. An anastomotic leak becomes apparent about four to seven days after surgery and is heralded by chills, fever, and abdominal pain. This occurs in anywhere from 1% to 12% of colon anastomoses depending upon the surgeon, patient, and type of operation. Some leaks are tiny and go away on their own. Others are large enough to permit stool and gas to leak freely into the abdominal cavity, and can result in death if not treated promptly. In the case of a small leak, withholding diet for a few days (usually with intravenous nutrition in hospital) may be all that is required. In the case of a serious leak, reoperation is mandatory. The anastomosis may have to be taken apart in this case or protected by placing a stoma in the bowel upstream (see Chapter 43 for a discussion of stomas). Subsequently, re-anastomosis or closure of the protective stoma may be attempted when the patient has fully recovered.

LATE POSTOPERATIVE COMPLICATIONS

Late postoperative complications include bowel obstruction and narrowing of the anastomosis (called *anastomotic stricture*). If a stoma is made, complications such as retraction or herniation of the stoma may develop.

Bowel obstruction results from scar tissue that forms in the abdomen cavity as a result of surgery. The scar tissue may constrict the bowel and block it.

Some degree of postoperative obstruction is common after major abdominal surgery and can happen from a few weeks to years later in as many as 20% of patients. Fortunately, most episodes of bowel obstruction from scar tissue are transient and no surgery is required.

Narrowing of the anastomosis is fairly common and usually requires either no treatment or only minor stretching of the anastomosis in the surgeon's office or the operating room. The presence of a narrowed anastomosis is most often indicated by an increasing difficulty to evacuate stool. Rates of anastomotic stricture vary from 5% to 20% in stapled anastomoses performed during anterior resection for a rectal cancer.

REDUCING THE COMPLICATION RATE

Patients may have some control over their own complication rate by their choice of surgeon and operation, and by modifying some of their own habits.

THE SURGEON

Most surgeons do not know their own complication rates, so it is essentially impossible for a patient to know them. Few surgeons keep track of their own complications in a form that can be updated and reviewed, and what information is known is not made public anywhere. Even a surgeon cannot judge another surgeon's surgical ability without spending time in the operating room with him or her.

Recommendations by friends tend to be based on the quality of the surgeon's bedside manner. Keep in mind that the best surgeons do not necessarily possess the warmest bedside manner. Some busy surgeons are not interested in being overly friendly with their patients, believing that a detached manner is the most efficient.

Your best method of finding a good surgeon is to work with your family physician to get a surgeon with special interest in colorectal surgery. The surgeon should be performing the type of operation that you need frequently, and should have a minimum of four years in surgical practice after completion of all training. If you can obtain this level of care, you have done well.

THE OPERATION

The operation ultimately chosen to deal with a cancer will depend upon the surgeon's preference and experience, the location, grade, and stage of the cancer along with the patient's wishes. In most cases, the type of operation is dictated by the location of the cancer and there is little controversy. In those cases of very low rectal cancers where there is some choice of procedure, each of these procedures will have a different complication rate. See Chapters 21 and 26 for a discussion of the choices of operations for low rectal cancer.

THE PATIENT

If you stop smoking, even for as little as a few weeks before surgery, you may reduce the elevated risk of postoperative lung complications that smokers experience. If you drink alcohol every day, wean yourself off it before the operation so there will be no problems with withdrawal symptoms in the postoperative phase. If you have significant tooth decay or a problem tooth, get it dealt with before surgery since tooth infections can increase the risk of postoperative lung infections. If you are diabetic, review your blood sugar management with your internist and have a plan to manage it optimally before and after surgery. Finally, for those who are overweight and are on a list for surgery several weeks away, a little weight loss can make the operation easier for the surgeon (although starving oneself before a major operation is not recommended).

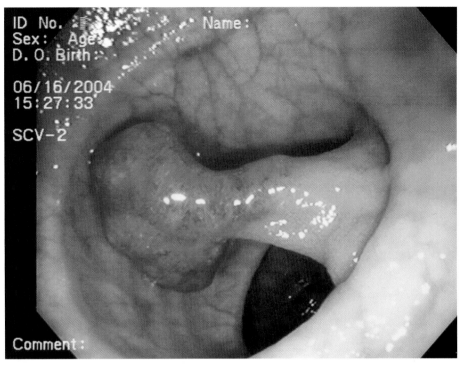

Figure a. *A large adenoma.*

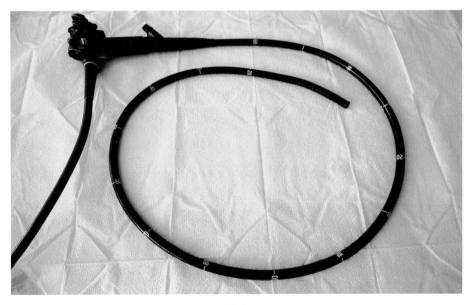

Figure b. *Colonoscope.*

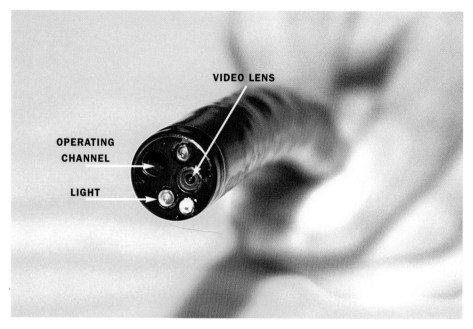

Figure c(i). *Tip of a colonoscope.*

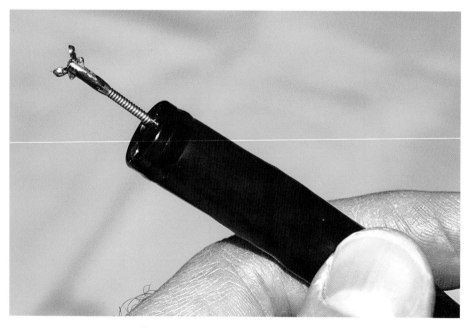

Figure c(ii). *Biopsy forcep (jaws open) projecting from the end of colonoscope operating channel.*

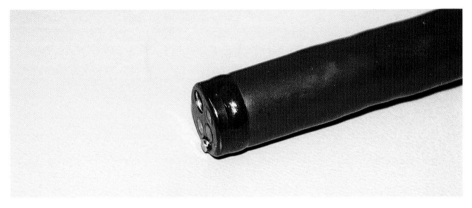

Figure d(i). *Colonoscope tip.*

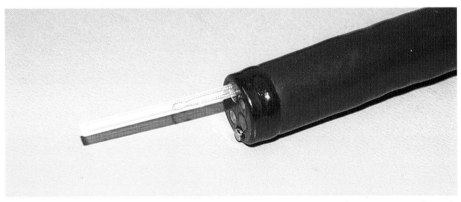

Figure d(ii). *Plastic sheath (containing polypectomy snare) projecting from operating channel.*

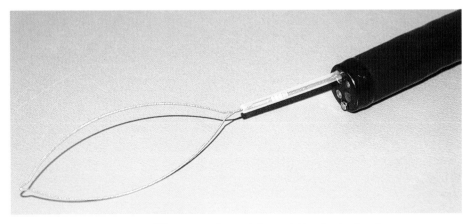

Figure d(iii). *Wire snare advanced from within plastic sheath.*

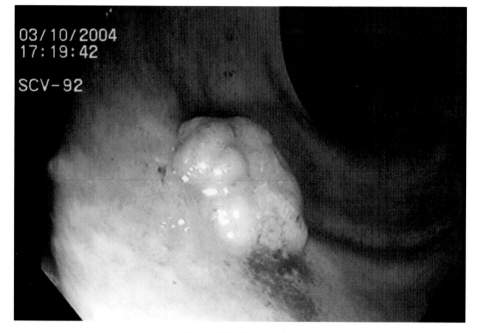

Figure e(i). *Colon polyp.*

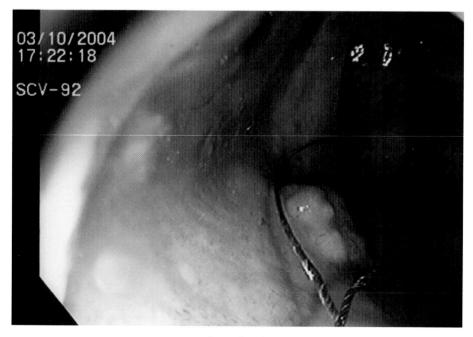

Figure e(ii). *Wire loop placed around the polyp.*

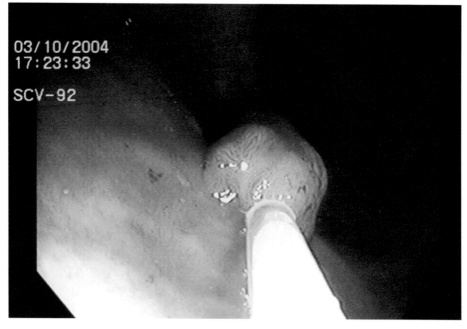

Figure e(iii). *Wire loop is tightened as plastic sheath is advanced.*

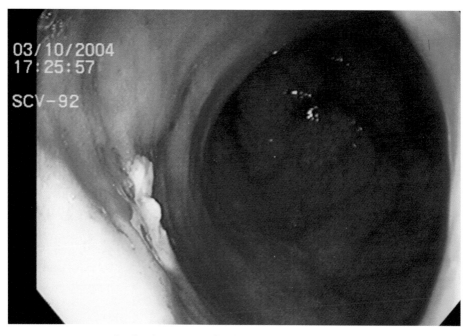

Figure e(iv). *Polyp has been removed—electrical current has sealed blood vessels.*

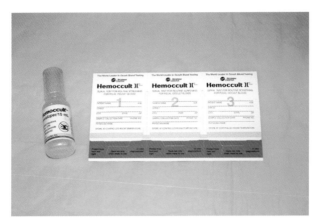

Figure f. *Three-panel kit tests stool for occult blood.*

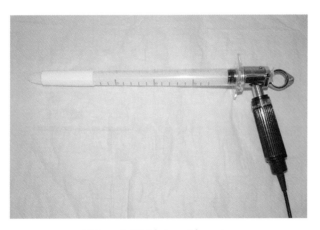

Figure g. *Rigid sigmoidoscope.*

HANDLE ⟶

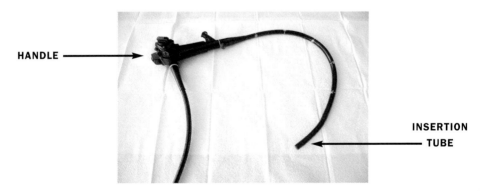

INSERTION TUBE

Figure h. *Flexible sigmoidoscope.*

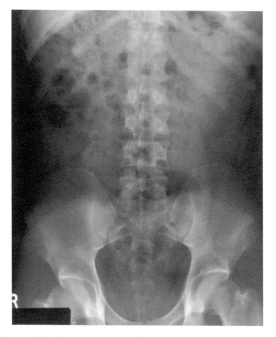

Figure i(i). *Plain abdominal X-ray—the colon is not seen.*

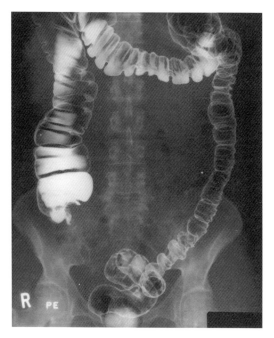

Figure i(ii). *Barium enema—barium makes the colon visible.*

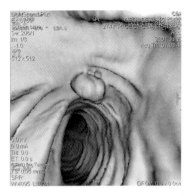

Figure j. *Polyp seen on virtual colonoscopy (colonography).*

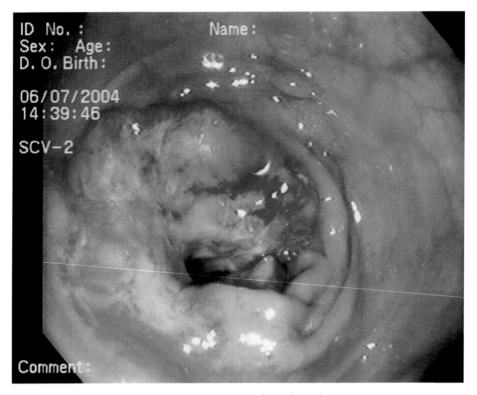

Figure k. *Colon cancer as seen through a colonoscope.*

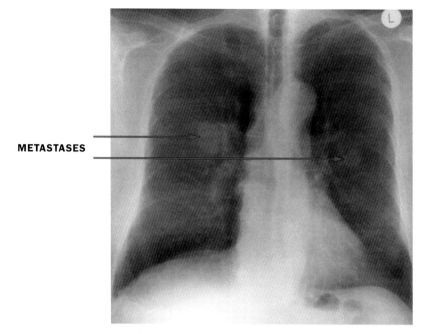

METASTASES

Figure l. *Chest X-ray showing cancer that has spread to the lungs.*

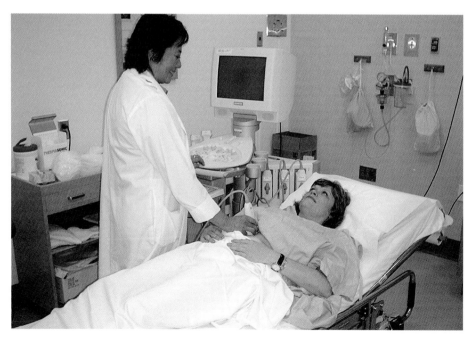

Figure m. *Undergoing abdominal ultrasound.*

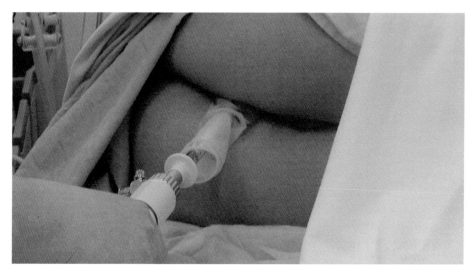

Figure n(i). *Performing endorectal ultrasound.*

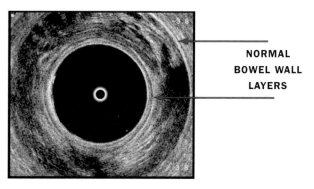

NORMAL
BOWEL WALL
LAYERS

Figure n(ii). *Normal endorectal ultrasound.*

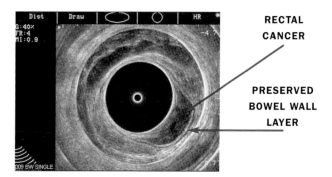

RECTAL
CANCER

PRESERVED
BOWEL WALL
LAYER

Figure n(iii). *Superficial rectal cancer, circular layers preserved.*

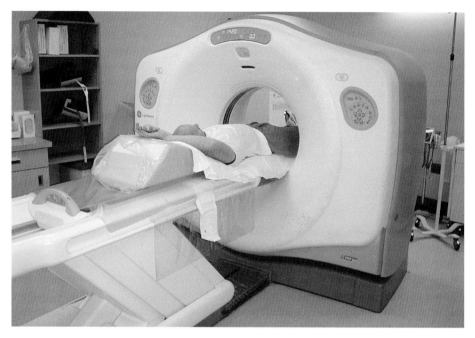

Figure o(i). *CT scanner.*

METASTASES

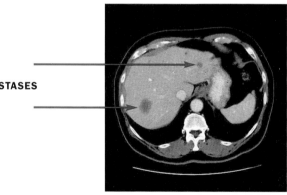

Figure o(ii). *CT scan "slice" shows metastases in liver.*

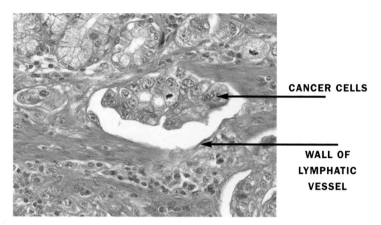

CANCER CELLS

WALL OF
LYMPHATIC
VESSEL

Figure p. *Clump of cancer cells within a lymphatic vessel.*

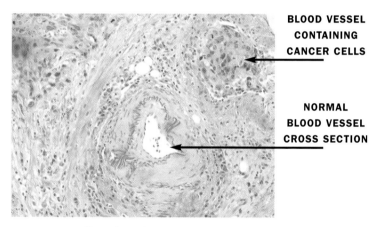

BLOOD VESSEL
CONTAINING
CANCER CELLS

NORMAL
BLOOD VESSEL
CROSS SECTION

Figure q. *Cancer cells within a blood vessel (vascular invasion).*

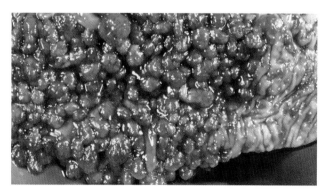

Figure r. *Hundreds of small adenomatous polyps in this FAP colon specimen.*

DEALING WITH A COMPLICATION

If you suffer a complication following surgery, should you let your original surgeon try to deal with it or should you "fire" him or her and get a new surgeon? We suspect that even Donald Trump would tell you that the best thing to do is let the original surgeon deal with it. He or she is already familiar with your case and generally knows best what is happening. Since complications are a fact of life in surgery, they do not necessarily mean the surgeon should be changed. Changing surgeons after the development of a complication would be appropriate only if there is reason to believe that there has been negligence on the part of the surgeon. This is rare.

In some cases, if the complication is an unusual one or particularly difficult to deal with, a surgeon will seek a second opinion from an experienced colleague. This can be taken as a sign of the surgeon's desire to obtain the best possible outcome for his patient rather than an indication of weakness or uncertainty. Such a review should be welcomed by the patient.

If you have had a complication and are concerned about the appropriateness of proposed management, it would not be out of line to request your surgeon to arrange a second opinion for you. A high quality surgeon will not resent this and a colleague will generally provide an honest opinion about what he or she would do in such a case irrespective of the workplace relationship with your attending surgeon.

11

SPECIAL SURGICAL CONSIDERATIONS

CHAPTER 24
MANAGING THE MALIGNANT POLYP

THE OBVIOUSLY MALIGNANT POLYP FOUND AT COLONOSCOPY

If, while performing a colonoscopy, the examiner concludes that a polyp is really a small cancer, he or she must make a decision about whether to attempt a polypectomy or not. An experienced colonoscopist can usually tell the difference between a benign polyp and a small cancer. The polyp that is primarily cancerous will look different and will feel much harder when probed by the polypectomy snare.

A basic principle of all cancer surgery is that cancers should be removed intact to prevent spillage of cancer cells into surrounding tissues. Leaving a small cancer in place is the most appropriate decision for the colonoscopist to make. A polypectomy could cut through the cancer, violating the rule that cancer should be removed in one piece. So, rather than doing a polypectomy, a tiny biopsy is taken to confirm the diagnosis and the patient is referred to a surgeon for assessment and probable removal of that segment of bowel.

THE BENIGN-LOOKING POLYP THAT TURNS OUT TO HAVE A PORTION OF CANCER WITHIN IT

The more common clinical situation is not the obviously cancerous polyp, but the benign-appearing polyp that has already been removed and, when examined microscopically by the pathologist, has a section of cancer within it. The question is, "What do we do now?"

WHAT ARE THE ODDS THAT SOME CANCER HAS BEEN LEFT BEHIND?

If the cut edge of the removed polyp shows cancer, it means that the chances are quite high that the cancer was cut through during the polypectomy and that not all of the cancer has been removed. In such cases something more needs to be done. Usually, surgery is necessary (see below). Fortunately, the more common situation is that the cancer in the polyp was entirely removed by polypectomy and there is no cancer at the cut edge. In this case, the key concern is the possibility that some of the cancer from the polyp had already spread to the lymph nodes adjacent to that segment of bowel before the polypectomy. If nothing further is done, the cancer left behind in those lymph nodes will grow and spread and ultimately be fatal to the patient. Therefore, in order to decide what to do next, the odds of metastatic spread to the adjacent lymph nodes (Figure 25) must be determined.

If one could determine that there were no involved lymph nodes in the case of a removed polyp that contained some cancer, then no further treatment beyond the polypectomy would be required. If, on the other hand, one could show that adjacent lymph nodes contained cancer, excision of that segment of bowel along with those adjacent lymph nodes would be mandatory unless the patient was unfit for such surgery or the cancer was already widespread.

If the site of the polyp was the rectum, endorectal ultrasound (see Chapter 13) may reveal suspicious-looking lymph nodes beside the rectum suggesting lymph node metastases. This finding would favor surgery. Conversely, the

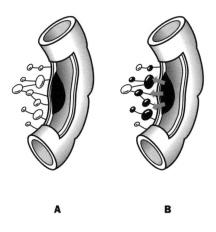

A   B

Figure 25. *Who has lymph node spread? It may be impossible to distinguish between patients who do not have cancer in the lymph nodes (A) and those who do (B).*

absence of such lymph nodes during an endorectal ultrasound examination would be reassuring. But in most cases, current testing methods are not good enough to determine the presence or absence of lymph node metastases unless they are large and obvious. Instead, we use statistical information based upon previous cases to predict the likelihood of lymph node involvement in a patient who has had a malignant polyp removed. A number of factors are taken into consideration to determine the probability of cancer in the lymph nodes. These include the following:

Has the actual focus of cancer been removed?

If the polypectomy snare cut through the focus of cancer rather than through the normal tissue beneath it, there is a problem. Pathologists can determine that the cancer has been cut through if the cancer cells come right up to the edge of the cut surface of the specimen. Edges are very important to pathologists. They study the edges of all cancer specimens microscopically to determine whether they are clear of cancer or not. If cancer cells are seen at the edge, one has to assume that the cancer cells adjacent to this cut edge are still in the patient. In such cases, the specimen is said to have an *incomplete resection margin*. Another way of saying this is that the margin is *not clear*, or the margin is *involved*. An adequate or clear resection margin has at least one mm ($^1/_{32}$ inch) of normal tissue at the cut edge.

To remedy the situation of an incomplete resection margin after polypectomy, one might consider redoing the colonoscopy to find the stalk of the polyp and try to take more of it in hopes of removing the remaining cancer tissue and getting a clear margin. If the polyp had a head and a stalk and part of the stalk is still left, this might be reasonable. But in most cases, the incomplete margin more often represents a deeply penetrating cancer and it is more prudent to remove that segment of bowel, along with its lymph nodes, at surgery. When a polypectomy has been correctly performed, but there is an incomplete resection margin, the likelihood of lymph node metastases is 30% to 48%.

What was the polyp itself like?

Certain characteristics of the size and shape of the polyp suggest the likelihood of lymph node metastases. Polyps less than 10 mm ($^1/_2$ inch) in diameter are more likely safe than bigger ones. Flat polyps of 10 mm or more that contain cancer are quite unsafe, with a positive lymph node incidence of 29%. The most troublesome polyp configuration is when the abnormality is actually a depression on the bowel wall rather than an abnormality sticking up from the lining. Depressed lesions of any size are associated with a 75% risk of lymph node involvement.

Where did the cancer lie within the polyp?

The closer the focus of cancer in a polyp lies to the actual bowel wall, the greater the likelihood of lymph node metastases and, therefore, the more sensible surgery becomes. The position of cancer within a polyp has been classified to reflect the likelihood of lymph node metastases. This classification is called Haggitt's classification (Figure 26).

If the polyp has a head and stalk, a determination is made as to whether the cancer is limited to the head of the polyp, or is in the stalk, or has penetrated to the base of the stalk. Cancers limited to the head of the polyp have a very low risk of lymph node metastases (Haggitt's level 1). The further down the polyp the cancer lies, the greater the risk of lymph node metastases; the risk reaching 15% if the base of the stalk is involved (Haggitt's level 4). Polyps that are flat and contain penetrating cancer are automatically considered Haggitt's level 4.

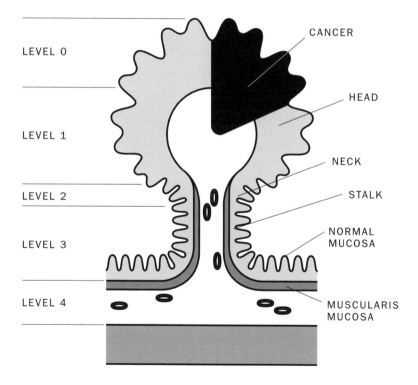

Figure 26. *Haggitt's classification. Useful for predicting the chance of lymph node metastases associated with a malignant polyp.*

What are the microscopic characteristics of the actual focus of cancer? Some cancer cells are more aggressive-looking under the microscope than others. The medical term for aggressive-looking cancer is *poorly differentiated* cancer. If the cancer cells in the polyp are poorly differentiated, there is a higher rate of lymph node metastases than if the cells are well differentiated.

If, under the microscope, the cancer cells appear to penetrate the lymphatic vessels or the blood vessels within the polyp, the cancer is revealing its ability to spread. The incidence of lymph node metastases when there is microscopic evidence of lymphatic vessel or blood vessel invasion is high (50%).

PUTTING IT ALL TOGETHER TO MAKE THE DECISION
ABOUT WHETHER SURGERY IS REQUIRED

In order to decide if additional surgery is required after a malignant polyp is removed, the physician must put together the information about the polyp and its cancer, its location in the bowel, the likelihood of there being lymph node metastases, whether there are other metastases found, the fitness of the patient for surgery, and the patient's treatment preferences.

If there are already metastases of cancer in the liver or lungs, removing the segment of bowel that contained the malignant polyp may not be of much value. Fortunately, in most cases of a malignant polyp, distant metastases are rare and the decision whether to operate is fairly straight-forward. If the polyp possesses any unsafe (unfavorable) features and the patient is well enough to tolerate surgery, the segment of bowel is usually removed. Unfavorable features would include any Haggitt's level 3 or 4 cancer, any cancer that shows venous or lymphatic invasion, any cancer that is at the resection margin (cut edge) of the polyp, and any poorly dif-ferentiated cancer. If there are no unfavorable features, the polypectomy alone is usually considered satisfactory treatment.

TWO SPECIAL MALIGNANT POLYP SITUATIONS

THE CASE OF THE MALIGNANT POLYP IN THE FRAIL PATIENT

In the case of the frail patient, the decision of whether to operate after removing a malignant polyp can be made somewhat easier by taking into account both the risk of surgery and adding that to the odds of lymph node involvement. If the chance of lymph node metastases is determined to be 10%, the operation has a 90% chance of not helping that person. If one considers that surgery cures only one-half of patients with lymph node metastases, the patient now faces a 5% chance of being helped by surgery and a 95% chance of having no benefit from surgery. If to that, one adds the risk of operation in a frail person, say 3% chance of death, we are now looking at a situation where the operation has a 2% chance of benefit versus a 98% chance of harm or no benefit. Therefore, unless the frail patient would otherwise be expected to have a substantial life expectancy, surgery would not be warranted.

THE CASE OF THE MALIGNANT POLYP LOW IN THE RECTUM

Some malignant polyps are so low in the rectum that aggressive surgical treatment would require compete removal of the sphincter muscles and permanent colostomy. Should the patient accept a colostomy or play the odds that all the cancer is gone? In this situation every relevant staging test assessing for distant metastases and rectal lymph nodes should be performed in order to determine whether surgery makes sense. In a patient who is otherwise well, if there are no distant metastases and there appear to be enlarged lymph nodes adjacent to the rectum, surgery is almost certainly the only rational choice. But sometimes no answers about the status of the lymph nodes can be gleaned by any test and the only certain way of knowing the lymph nodes are adequately treated is by doing the operation and removing them (with the rectum). A second opinion from a respected specialist should be sought before the final decision is made. If the choice is for surgery, the patient and the surgeon must be prepared to be satisfied that they made the right choice even if the pathologist's study of the resected specimen later reveals that the lymph nodes do not contain cancer. Provided that patients in this situation are psychologically prepared for whatever the results are, they will be comforted by knowing they made a choice for life and that, given all the information available at the time, it was the correct choice regardless of the outcome.

CHAPTER 25
LAPAROSCOPIC SURGERY FOR
COLORECTAL CANCER

Unlike traditional surgery that requires a large incision to enter the abdomen, *laparoscopic surgery* uses a series of small (often less than 1.5 cm [$^1/_2$ inch]) incisions. A specially designed video camera is passed through one of the small incisions into the abdomen to permit the surgical team to see into the abdomen. Grasping and dissecting instruments are passed through the other small incisions. By watching the video monitor, the surgeon uses the dissecting and grasping instruments to manipulate the bowel and perform the operation.

Laparoscopic surgery was first widely used by gynecologists to avoid large incisions when assessing the fallopian tubes and ovaries and for performing small operations such as tubal ligation (to prevent pregnancy). Laparoscopy became much more widely known when it was discovered that it was an ideal way to remove the gallbladder. It is now quite rare for a gallbladder to be removed through a traditional incision in North America. The explosive growth of laparoscopic gallbladder surgery came when it was found that the recovery time was substantially shorter than after the traditional incision operation. Traditional surgery gallbladder patients used to stay in hospital for a week, whereas laparoscopic surgery gallbladder patients began going home the next day or even the same day. The cost savings of reduced hospital days and rapid return to work accelerated the acceptance of laparoscopic gallbladder surgery beyond that of any previous operation.

Given the clear success of laparoscopic surgery for the gallbladder, it was natural for surgeons to try the laparoscopic approach for many different operations, including colorectal operations. For many general surgery procedures, laparoscopy is clearly beneficial. But for colorectal procedures, reviews were, initially, not very favorable. It was discovered that laparoscopic surgery for intestinal or colorectal cases was much more difficult than it was for gallbladder surgery. The gallbladder is easier to operate on because it is a fixed target, firmly attached to the liver. The colon, however, is a moving target due to much looser attachments, and in most areas it is covered by the very mobile and squirming small intestine. Establishing a solid yet gentle hold of the colon required to perform the surgery while, at the same time, preventing the small intestine from sliding into the field and obscuring the view requires great experience. Generally, most surgeons felt that they had neither the patience nor the amount of operating time necessary to devote to learning the technique, and they have continued to use the traditional approach for most types of colorectal surgery.

There are two other reasons why laparoscopic colorectal surgery has not been widely adopted. First, unlike in the case of gallbladder surgery, it has taken some time to show that laparoscopic colorectal surgery reduces recovery time when compared to traditional colorectal surgery. Second, it was not known whether operating laparoscopically was as good a way of dealing with a cancer as the traditional open-incision method. Strange and disturbing reports of colon cancer metastases appearing in the tiny instrument stab wounds some months after laparoscopic surgery initially caused a great deal of concern.

Recently, innovations designed to make the procedure easier for the colorectal surgeon have included a hybrid (*laparoscopic-assisted*) operation where the surgeon makes one larger incision through which a special port is inserted that allows the surgeon to pass a single hand into the abdomen. The rest of the operation is done as a laparoscopic procedure except that now the surgeon can grasp the colon with a hand or move the small intestine out of the way as he or she would normally do. This greatly simplifies the procedure, but whether this will be the norm for colorectal cancer surgery in the future is not yet known.

In May of 2004, the first major credible comparison of standard operation versus laparoscopic-assisted operation for colon cancer was published. The study included 872 patients from a total of 48 institutions. Patients were followed for an average of 4.5 years from surgery. Researchers found that the rate of recurrence of cancer and the overall survival rate appeared to be the same in both the traditional surgery group and the laparoscopic-assisted group. The complication rate in both groups was the same. Patients recovered somewhat faster in the laparoscopic group, leaving hospital a day earlier and using pain medications for fewer days.

This study shows the promise of laparoscopic-assisted surgery for colon cancer and it is likely that the procedure will soon become more widely available. However, a couple of important points need to be made about the study. Firstly, the surgeons involved in this study were highly trained, selected, and motivated (they had to send in video tapes of their skills in order to be selected to take part!). It remains to be seen if laparoscopic surgery for colon cancer, when undertaken by a wider range of surgeons, will yield as good a result given that the benefits documented in the study are somewhat modest. Secondly, it should be understood that these results have been achieved in patients with colon cancer, not rectal cancer. Rectal cancer is more difficult surgery and whether a laparoscopic approach is suitable remains to be determined.

Traditional and even laparoscopic operations for rectal cancer require that the cancer-bearing rectum, or a portion of the rectum, be removed through the abdomen. These procedures are substantial and involve a considerable period of pain for the patient. Moreover, the removal of a portion of the rectum can damage surrounding tissue and may leave the patient with frequent or urgent bowel movements, altered control of stool, changes in sexual function, or other problems. *Localized treatments* are those directed at the cancer through the anus. They are designed to destroy or remove the rectal cancer without the need for major abdominal surgery and its drawbacks. In some cases of very low rectal cancer, localized treatment can prevent a colostomy. Localized treatment forms include:

- ► Surgical removal of the cancer through the anus rather than through the abdomen (trans-anal excision).
- ► Radiation of the cancer instead of surgery.

> ► Burning, freezing, laser treatment, or other ways of attempting to destroy the cancer through the anus.

WHY ARE LOCALIZED TREATMENTS USED ONLY RARELY?

Everyone agrees that these treatments are more easily tolerated than surgery through the abdomen, and they may be just as good at eradicating a small rectal cancer as the big operations. However, there are few patients for whom they are suited. The reason for this is the concern that the cancer itself may no longer be localized. It may have spread to the adjacent lymph nodes where it is beyond the reach of the localized treatment. None of the localized treatment options includes removal of lymph nodes. Accordingly, localized treatment is generally restricted to patients for whom traditional surgery is too risky, or patients with very early, superficial cancers that are unlikely to have spread to the lymph nodes but would require an abdominoperineal operation with permanent colostomy otherwise.

Most types of localized treatment are no longer considered valid. These include electrocoagulation therapy, cryotherapy (directly freezing the cancer with a probe), and laser therapy. While radiation therapy does have the potential of being useful as a sole treatment in some cases, it is rarely used in this way and is more often given as a treatment in addition to trans-anal excision of the cancer.

TRANS-ANAL EXCISION: WHAT IS IT AND WHO SHOULD HAVE IT?

Trans-anal excision is an operation in which the surgeon cuts out a small rectal cancer though the anus instead of through the abdomen. A retractor is placed into the anus in order for the surgeon to adequately see the cancer (Figure 27). A cautery (electrical burning) device is used to cut around the cancer and remove it along with a portion of normal surrounding tissue. The defect in the rectum is then sewn closed.

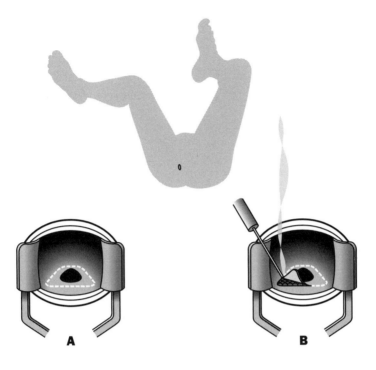

Figure 27. *Trans-anal excision of a small, low, superficial rectal cancer.*

For the rare patient with a rectal cancer that is small and superficial and has no "adverse" features, trans-anal excision, when combined with radiotherapy, gives results similar to those obtained by traditional operations. In order to be initially treated with trans-anal excision, a patient's cancer must meet all of the following conditions:

▶ It is not deeply penetrating (the cancer is a T1 or T2 cancer—see Chapter 15).

▶ It has a biopsy that shows mild microscopic features, as follows:

• Well differentiated or moderately well differentiated cancer.

• No evidence of lymphatic or vascular invasion.

• No evidence that it is "mucus-producing" (mucus-producing cancers being more aggressive).

In addition, once the procedure has been done, the resection margin of the fully removed specimen is examined and found to be clear of cancer (that is, the entire cancer appears to have been removed). If the resection margins are not clear, a re-operation will be required, and this will usually be the traditional operation that would otherwise have been done.

The rates of local recurrence for T1 cancers following trans-anal excision range from 1% to 15% if treated by surgery alone or 0% to 6% if radiation therapy is added afterward. For T2 cancers, local recurrence rates range from 10% to over 40% with surgery alone or 7% to 14% if radiotherapy is added. For T1 and T2 cancers after local excision, the five-year recurrence-free survival is about 85%, with or without radiotherapy.

It is essential to have careful follow-up evaluation after localized treatment. In fact, it is more important than after conventional surgery because a local recurrence can still be treated by traditional surgical operations with a reasonable hope of cure if a recurrence is identified early.

Follow-up assessment takes the form of regular digital and rigid sigmoidoscopy inspection of the excision site. This should be done by the surgeon who did the operation. Examinations should be performed every three months during the first two years, then every six months for the next three years. At five years, if there is no sign of trouble, the patient is likely cured, but will require regular screening of the entire colon because of the potential risk for other colorectal cancers (patients who have had one colorectal cancer are at increased risk for developing another one.

Cancer may be called *advanced* if it has grown very deeply into its original (primary) site or if it has spread (metastasized) to other sites. Advanced cancers may be divided into two main groups: those that are potentially curable by surgery, and those that are not. A cancer that is potentially curable by surgery is one that can be removed with no obvious cancer left behind. In such cases, even though surgery may be extensive, there is still the hope for cure. A cancer that is not potentially curable by surgery means that obvious or presumed cancer tissue would be left behind at the completion of an operation. The reasons why all cancer may not be removable is that the cancer may have spread into body parts that cannot be sacrificed, or because the pattern of spread suggests that there are other areas of spread that cannot be seen.

ADVANCED CANCER POTENTIALLY CURABLE BY SURGERY

A DEEPLY PENETRATING CANCER

A cancer that has grown deeply into its *primary site* (*locally advanced*) may penetrate through the rectum or colon and grow into an adjacent organ. Rectal cancer may grow into the vagina, uterus, bladder, or prostate gland. A colon cancer may also grow into the tissue adjacent to the colon, such as the small intestine or stomach.

One of the most important principles of cancer surgery is that a cancer must be removed in one piece. If a cancer is fractured during surgery, malignant cells may break off from the fracture site and spread the cancer in that area (called a *local recurrence*). Thus, if the cancer is found to be growing into an adjacent organ, the surgeon must attempt to remove that organ along with the cancerous segment of bowel, all in one piece. This concept of removing more than one organ type in one piece with the cancer attached is called *en bloc resection*. As an example, the uterus may have to be removed en bloc with a rectal cancer in a case where the rectal cancer has penetrated into the uterus (Figure 28). While this kind of surgery may be technically challenging, there have been many well-documented cures following en bloc resection.

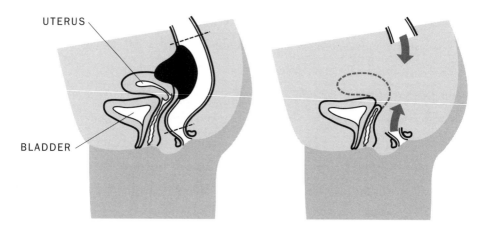

Figure 28. *En bloc removal of a rectal cancer and the uterus in one piece. The top of the vagina will be closed and the bowel sewn or stapled together.*

Patients usually do well after the removal of the uterus, fallopian tubes, or ovaries as part of an en bloc resection since most affected patients are already beyond menopause. Similarly, removal of a portion of the stomach, liver, upper portion of the urinary bladder, or the spleen is usually tolerated well. The most difficult situation occurs when the lower bladder or prostate gland becomes involved with a deeply penetrating rectal cancer. To remove these areas en bloc with a rectal cancer, the entire urinary system in the pelvis must be removed, and an opening on the abdominal wall (a urinary stoma) created for the passage of urine. This is rarely done for rectal cancer. It is a very big operation and results have been discouraging.

Obviously, one would never consider this type of heroic operation unless meticulous preliminary staging (see Chapter 13) of the patient's cancer revealed no evidence of cancer spread beyond this area. It is one thing to suffer through such a major procedure with the hope of a cure. It is quite another, and completely unfair, to put someone through such an ordeal if the chance for cure is low or nonexistent.

Preoperative radiation may play a role in preparing a locally advanced rectal cancer for surgery by weakening its attachments to surrounding structures of the pelvis (see Chapter 18).

WHEN THERE ARE METASTASES

The question of whether metastases should be surgically removed requires careful assessment of the individual case. Each situation is unique. Removing metastases is always a question of odds since the cancer has already proven it has the ability to spread, and there may already be other, invisible metastases that are just beginning to grow, in addition to the obvious one (or ones) that the surgeon is contemplating removing. When considering surgical removal, careful staging is performed to determine whether the cancer has spread to one site or to multiple sites.

The single metastasis

Provided the patient is in reasonable physical condition and the primary (original) site of cancer seems to have been removed favorably, most surgeons will attempt to remove a single metastasis, almost irrespective of where it is (Figure 29). If the single metastasis is the only identifiable site of cancer spread, the patient stands a reasonable chance of being cured by its surgical removal. A biphasic CT scan is probably the most useful and accurate way to look for colorectal metastases in the liver. MRI does not usually add much to the CT information.

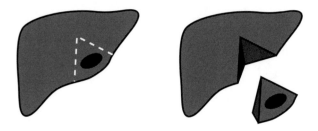

Figure 29. *Excision of a solitary colorectal cancer liver metastasis.*

The five-year survival rates (similar to cure rates) of patients with completely removed single liver metastases from colorectal cancer range from 18% to 46% in different studies.

Why aren't all single metastases curable? The problem is that where there is one metastasis, there are likely to be more; perhaps as yet too small to be seen. It is like the story of the solitary horseman that appears on a hill, followed by another solitary horseman, and another, until the entire hillside is covered by "solitary" horsemen. We always hope that the metastasis we see is the only one present, but this is often not the case. Nonetheless, most surgeons will attempt to remove a single metastasis provided the patient appears able to tolerate the surgery.

Multiple metastases

The number of surgical success stories diminishes as the number of metastases increases. Whereas it is almost always reasonable to operate on a single metastasis, the presence of two or three suggests a much less favorable situation, and when there are more than three, surgery is difficult to justify. The potential harm, suffering, and time in hospital away from family, do not support aggressive surgery when cancer has spread to more than three sites.

Who should operate on metastases?

If your cancer has spread, it is a good idea to seek a second opinion from a surgeon experienced in dealing with advanced cancer when considering whether to undergo attempted surgical removal of the metastases. This type of surgery is best done by surgeons affiliated with major cancer referral centers who deal with this problem frequently and who have the back-up of a full range of surgical and medical specialties and care units. Surgery of this kind is not for the surgeon in a small hospital who deals with these cases infrequently.

Other ways of dealing with liver metastases

Radiofrequency ablation is a new form of treatment in which alternating current is passed through the tumor, generating heat that destroys the tumor. A probe is inserted into the tumor, either through the abdominal wall or at laparotomy. For this treatment to be useful, patients must have just a few tumors in the liver (usually not more than five), each of which must be relatively small in size (usually not more than 5 cm in diameter). Early results of this treatment are promising.

ADVANCED CANCER NOT CURABLE BY SURGERY

LOCALLY ADVANCED—NOT REMOVABLE

It is unusual for a colon or rectal cancer to be so advanced that it cannot be removed surgically. Many rectal cancers may at first be found to be tethered or penetrating deeper tissues, but these are generally still removable. They are made more easily removable by preoperative radiotherapy (see Chapter 18) as it seems to loosen the tumor attachments. Such radiation treatment, when combined with chemotherapy, may also improve surgical cure rates.

More often, the patient who may be deemed unsuitable for removal of the primary site of cancer is the one with widespread incurable metastases. In such cases, a heroic operation to get a deeply penetrating primary tumor out no longer makes sense. Still, if the primary cancer is a rectal cancer, it is often worth removing, even when there are metastases. The reason for this is that if the patient lives nine to 18 months, a deeply penetrating rectal cancer may begin to cause serious pain well before the patient succumbs from the metastases. So, as a basic principle, only in cases where metastases are truly widespread and life expectancy is short is the primary cancer left in place.

For some other types of cancer, it makes sense to have at least parts of the cancer removed if surgeons cannot get it all out. This is called *debulking* a cancer. In essence surgeons remove what they can and leave the rest behind, hoping to add some time to the patient's remaining life. Unfortunately, debulking is not something that is done with colorectal cancer since it rarely improves survival and may lead to bleeding and other complications that impair the quality of the patient's remaining time.

METASTASES PRESENT AND NUMEROUS—NOT CURABLE

If there are numerous metastases present, the patient cannot be cured and removal of the metastases is usually not undertaken. A situation in which there are more than five metastases is generally considered incurable by most surgeons.

Sometimes a surgeon will open a patient's abdomen for a colorectal cancer operation and unexpectedly find that the lining membrane of the abdominal cavity is studded with tiny seed-like deposits of colorectal cancer. This situation is known as *carcinomatosis peritoneii*. The peritoneum is the name of the membrane lining the abdominal cavity and *carcinomatosis* refers to the diffuse seeding of the peritoneum by cancer. Carcinomatosis is incurable. Whether the surgeon goes ahead with the operation as planned (to get the primary cancer out) will depend upon the extent of the carcinomatosis, the status of the primary cancer, and the general condition of the patient. If the carcinomatosis is not extensive and the patient is in reasonable condition, the operation may go ahead as planned. It will not be curative, but it may minimize future problems, such as bowel obstruction from the cancer. On the other hand, if the carcinomatosis is extensive and the cancer is difficult to remove in a patient who is frail and not expected to live long, the operation should be modified to provide some temporary relief, or abandoned altogether.

12

PROGNOSIS AFTER SURGERY

CHAPTER 28
ASSESSING THE SURGICAL SPECIMEN

The pathologist will carefully assess the cancerous part removed during surgery to glean important information about the quality of the surgery, the stage of the cancer, prognosis, and the requirement for additional treatment. This assessment includes both visual inspection of the specimen and microscopic examination of representative pieces of the specimen.

VISUAL INSPECTION

Looking at the specimen with the naked eye can tell the pathologist quite a lot about the cancer and the skill of the surgeon. Is this cancer small and limited or does it seem advanced? Does the cancer appear to be completely contained within the specimen? Has the specimen been removed with optimal technique, ensuring the best possible outcome?

SIZE

By carefully feeling the specimen and cancer, the pathologist will discover the size of the primary cancer. Although not always the case, smaller cancers are generally easier to remove intact, are associated with a lower likelihood of lymph node metastases, and tend to result in a better overall prognosis.

DEPTH OF PENETRATION

Visual inspection will also indicate whether the cancer has penetrated through the wall of the bowel. Cancer feels harder than normal tissue and it looks whitish-gray, different from the red or pink normal tissues, so it can be readily identified on the outside wall of the specimen if it has penetrated through. Cancer that has penetrated through the specimen to appear on the outside of the specimen has exposed itself to the lining of the abdominal cavity, so the possibility exists that cells have already broken off from the cancer and seeded the abdominal cavity. Thus, such full thickness penetration is associated with a higher incidence of recurrence in the abdomen and a correspondingly worsened prognosis. Full thickness penetration is something that the surgeon cannot do anything about since it has occurred prior to surgery. All that can be done at the time of surgery is to try to protect the abdominal cavity from further contamination by covering or otherwise containing the cancerous segment of bowel during the operation.

LYMPH NODE METASTASES

The presence of lymph node metastases may be obvious to the pathologist when examining the specimen since cancerous nodes are often larger or firmer than normal. The pathologist will make careful note of the total number of lymph nodes and their location relative to the cancer. The lymph nodes will then be removed from the specimen for microscopic examination.

QUALITY OF THE SPECIMEN

In the past, surgeons would often open the cancer specimen at a side table in the operating room to demonstrate the cancer to medical students and resident staff. This is no longer considered appropriate in view of our improved understanding of the importance of the quality of specimen as an indicator of a patient's outcome. Leading pathologists now generally insist on receiving the specimen in an intact state in order to more accurately audit the cancer and the quality of the specimen.

The pathologist will check to see if there are any holes in the specimen, which would indicate that the bowel segment was torn or accidentally entered during its removal. If so, cancer cells may have escaped into the patient's pelvis. The pathologist will also check to see if the cut ends (margins) of the specimen of bowel are far enough away from the cancer so that the cancer was completely removed, or if the surgeon cut the bowel too close to the cancer.

In the case of a colon cancer, pathologists check to see if enough lymph nodes have been removed with the specimen. Patients with specimens containing fewer than seven lymph nodes have a worse outcome than patients whose specimens contained more lymph nodes. The reason for this is not entirely clear. It may indicate that the operation was less extensive or performed less expertly. Perhaps the cancerous lymph nodes have been left in the patient. In some cases, there just are not that many nodes even after an adequate operation. Importantly, an inadequate number of lymph nodes means that the pathologist is limited in his or her ability to accurately assess whether the cancer has spread to the lymph nodes since there are not enough to examine. This means that the patient may be *understaged*. Understaged patients might not be recommended to have certain postoperative treatments that would otherwise benefit them had their true stage been determined.

In the case of a rectal cancer, the new TME (total mesorectal excision) method of removing the rectal cancer specimen demands a high degree of exactness from the surgeon (see Chapter 21 for details). The mesorectum contains the lymph nodes and must be removed with the rectum as an intact package of fat and lymph nodes with its surrounding membrane unharmed (see Chapter 1). It has been found that when the pathologist works closely with the surgeon to audit and record the quality of the surgical specimen, patient results improve dramatically. The pathologist will grade the status of the mesorectum that is attached to the back of the rectal cancer specimen. This grading is a strong stimulus for surgeons to perfect their surgical technique.

MICROSCOPIC EXAMINATION

Once a colorectal cancer specimen has been carefully photographed and examined visually, it must be prepared for microscopic assessment (Figures 30 and 31). The front and back of the specimen are painted with ink to permit their identification under the microscope. The specimen is then placed in formaldehyde for a minimum of 72 hours, which embalms the specimen so that it can be safely examined without risk of spoiling. It is then thinly sliced into three to five mm ($^1/_8$ inch) slices from two cm ($^3/_4$ inch) below the cancer to two cm above. The slices are photographed as a valuable demonstration of the quality of the surgery. The pathologist looks at these cross sections with a naked eye and then cuts several blocks of cancer tissue for assessment under the microscope. The blocks are embedded in paraffin and then thinly sliced for viewing under a microscope. The key microscopic features that the pathologist looks for are the grade of the cancer, whether the cancer is contained within the specimen, how deeply it has penetrated, and whether the cancer has invaded into lymphatic vessel, lymph nodes, or blood vessels.

CANCER GRADE (MICROSCOPIC ASSESSMENT)

Colorectal cancers vary in how aggressively they grow and spread. One way of determining how aggressively a cancer will behave is to assess the appearance of its cells under the microscope. Based on the appearance, the pathologist gives the cancer an aggressiveness grade. In most cases, there will have been a biopsy (tissue sample) of the cancer prior to surgery so there will be

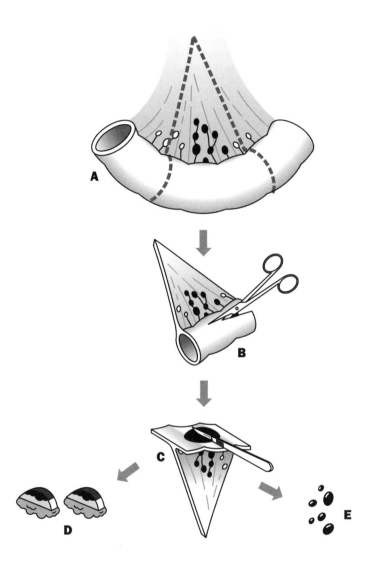

Figure 30. *Preparing the specimen 1.*

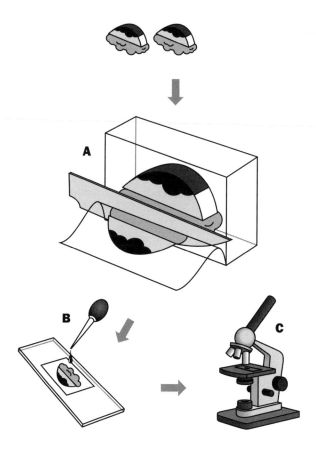

Figure 31. *Preparing the specimen 2.*

some preliminary indication of the grade. The pathologist will perform the same assessment on the surgical specimen, with the added advantage of having much more tissue to assess and so a greater likelihood of determining the grade accurately. The features used to determine grade include cell size and shape, orientation of the cells, and the ability to stain certain colors when dyes are placed on them.

A number of grading systems, each with its own vocabulary, are used to describe the grade of a cancer. The simplest is the *high grade/low grade* system in which a microscopically aggressive-looking cancer is called a *high-grade cancer*, while a less aggressive-looking cancer is called a *low-grade cancer*. A cancer of intermediate appearance is called an *average-grade cancer*.

Another common grading system is the *differentiation system*. It is based on the understanding that a normal cell is a differentiated cell. Normal cells are differentiated from the original cells of a human embryo. Cancer cells look, microscopically, more like primitive cells of the embryo, and so are called undifferentiated. A cancer made up of poorly differentiated cells is one which has cells that appear particularly primitive. A *poorly differentiated cancer* would be expected to behave aggressively. It would be equivalent to a high-grade cancer. A *well differentiated cancer* would appear less primitive under the microscope, and would be expected to be easier to cure, all things being equal. An average-grade cancer in the differentiation system is called *moderately differentiated cancer* (see Table 7).

TABLE 7. MICROSCOPIC CANCER GRADES— HOW TERMS COMPARE.

LEAST AGGRESSIVE	AVERAGE	MOST AGGRESSIVE
Low-grade	Medium-grade	High-grade
Well differentiated	Moderately differentiated	Poorly differentiated

DEPTH OF PENETRATION (NAKED EYE AND MICROSCOPIC ASSESSMENT)

Colorectal cancer develops from the inside (lining) layer of the bowel. As it grows, it penetrates deeper into the bowel wall, and ultimately may grow right through the bowel wall. Thus, depth of penetration provides information about the stage of the cancer. Is it very superficial (just in the lining)? Does it penetrate into the bowel wall but not all the way through? Does it penetrate all the way through and appear on the outside of the bowel? These important findings permit the pathologist to accurately stage the patient's cancer, determine prognosis, and provide data for decisions about appropriateness of additional treatment following surgery.

QUALITY OF THE MARGIN (NAKED EYE AND MICROSCOPIC ASSESSMENT)

In order for surgery to cure a colorectal cancer, all known cancer must be removed. If the margin of the specimen reveals cancer at its edge, either visibly or microscopically, there is said to have been an *incomplete excision*. In such situations, recurrence of the cancer in that same area is likely. In fact, if cancer is seen microscopically as close as one mm ($^{1}/_{16}$ inch) from a cut edge, it is considered to be incompletely excised.

LYMPHATIC INVASION (MICROSCOPIC ASSESSMENT)

Lymph nodes are examined microscopically to see if they contain cancer. The location of each of the nodes relative to the location of the cancer in the specimen will be noted, since a cancerous node farther from the cancer may suggest a worse prognosis than one closer to the cancer. In addition, lymphatic vessels within the specimen are examined to see if there is any evidence of invasion of the lympatic vessels by cancer cells (Figure p, color section).

VASCULAR INVASION (MICROSCOPIC ASSESSMENT)

The pathologist looks carefully at the microscopic blood vessels in the specimen. In more aggressive cancers, one can sometimes see evidence of cancer cells invading the blood vessels (*vascular invasion*). Vascular invasion (Figure q, color section) by cancer suggests that there has been a breach of the circulatory system and that there is a higher probability that the cancer may have spread, by means of the blood vessels, to other parts of the body.

ADDITIONAL STAGING INFORMATION PROVIDED TO THE PATHOLOGIST BY THE SURGEON

Once the pathologist has visually inspected and then microscopically assessed the specimen, he or she has a clear picture of the cancer within that specific piece of tissue. To this information is added any additional findings that the surgeon might have noticed during the operation. The critical element is whether the surgeon detected any evidence of additional colorectal cancer anywhere else in the abdomen. If so, a biopsy will almost certainly have been taken of the suspicious area by the surgeon during the operation. The pathologist will assess this biopsy microscopically and if it contains colorectal cancer cells, the patient has a metastasis.

Prognosis is a forecast of outcome. In the case of cancer treatment, it refers to the likelihood of being cured. An individual's prognosis is based upon the stage and grade of the cancer. Because colorectal cancer rarely recurs after more than five years, patients who reach the five-year mark (after treatment) are deemed to have been cured. For this reason, prognosis is described as the chances of surviving five years or five-year survival. In other words, a patient with a projected "75% five-year survival" would have a 75% chance of living five years after treatment (and would likely be cured at that point).

WHY FIVE-YEAR SURVIVAL FIGURES MAY BE MISLEADING

It would be simple to list the five-year survival figures for each cancer stage and allow you to find your stage on the table and read off the chances of being well in five years. However, it doesn't quite work that way.

First, no two patients are alike, yet when physicians determine the cancer stage of any person, patients are forced into an artificial similarity. There are still many personal characteristics of each individual and each cancer that cannot be taken into account by any staging system. This leaves room for some individuals to have different outcomes from others in their group.

Second, survival figures are based on how the disease progresses in many individuals, not just one or two. Large numbers are necessary in order to provide an average performance among a group of people who have many differences. Five-year survival numbers are useful for predicting what can be expected for 100 cancer patients with a specific stage. Thus, a five-year survival rate of 70% means that of 100 patients with that particular stage of cancer, 70 would be expected to survive five years and likely cured, and 30 would be expected to develop a recurrence and die of the disease. No one can say ahead of time that any particular patient will fall into the more or less fortunate group. Physicians can quote the odds, but only time can reveal what will happen to any particular individual.

FIVE-YEAR SURVIVAL FIGURES

The following general five-year survival ratings, related to stage (see Chapter 15) are quoted in the literature:

STAGE 0   97% of patients with this stage are expected to live five years and likely be cured.

STAGE I   96%

STAGE II   87%

STAGE III   55%–60% if one to three lymph nodes are cancerous

33% if four or more lymph nodes are cancerous

STAGE IV   2%–5%

Overall, the five-year survival rate for colorectal cancer, if all patients are put into one group, is slightly less than 50%. These figures do not reflect the improvements resulting from recent changes in chemotherapy and radiation and may not reflect the newer surgical procedures for rectal cancer. Such treatment is projected to increase survival figures by 15% to 17%. It must also be kept in mind that poorly differentiated cancers (see Chapter 28) may have a somewhat worse prognosis than the more common moderately or moderately well differentiated cancers.

WHAT ABOUT INCURABLE CANCERS?

Some cases of colorectal cancer are simply not curable. These are the cases in which there are numerous metastases or deep inoperable penetration at the site of the primary cancer. It is only fair for a physician to respond truthfully to a patient who wishes to know how long he or she can expect to live. In such cases, most physicians have been proven wrong or have heard of their colleagues being proven wrong enough times that they are reluctant to answer this question. However, for those patients who need to make realistic plans for their own and their family's future, some indication of life-expectancy is important. An average of 18 months is what can be expected by most patients with incurable colorectal cancer.

HOW AM I DOING?

Waiting five years to know if one is cured can be an enormous burden. What are the odds of cure at two or three years after colorectal cancer surgery? It is useful to know that 75% of colorectal cancer recurrences will occur within the first two years following surgical treatment. Therefore, those over two years without any evidence of recurrence are increasingly likely to have a good outcome.

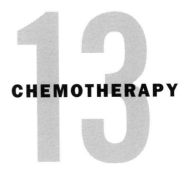

13

CHEMOTHERAPY

CHAPTER 30
WHAT IS CHEMOTHERAPY
AND HOW IS IT GIVEN?

Chemotherapy means the use of any drug or medication to treat disease. For example, antibiotics are a type of chemotherapy. Today, however, the word chemotherapy has come to refer specifically to the drugs that are used for treating cancer. There are dozens of different chemotherapy (anticancer) drugs. Because they work in different ways, several may be given at once (called *combination chemotherapy*).

The advantage of chemotherapy is that it travels in the blood stream, reaching cancer cells that may be in distant organs, away from the site of surgery or radiotherapy. In contrast, both surgery and radiotherapy are localized and target one area only.

THE USES OF CHEMOTHERAPY

Chemotherapy is used in two ways in treating colorectal cancer:

- ► Just before or just after cancer is surgically removed. When it is used this way it may be given before or after surgery and may or may not be combined with radiotherapy.

► When surgery cannot eliminate the cancer.

"BUT I'VE HEARD HORROR STORIES ABOUT CHEMOTHERAPY!"

Chemotherapy has a bad name due to the severe side effects patients used to experience when these drugs were first being developed. Because of these problems, a number of new drugs have since been developed that control or eliminate many of these side effects. They are given at the same time as the chemotherapy drugs, improving the patient's well-being while the chemotherapy goes to work on the cancer cells.

Changes in appearance, such as hair loss, also contribute to the dread of chemotherapy. Although disturbing, these changes are temporary (see Chapter 34).

Fear also stems from patients not having a clear idea *why* chemotherapy is being given. If chemotherapy is recommended as a part of your treatment, it is important for you to understand clearly the reasons for it or to ask the following questions:

► Why is the oncologist suggesting it?

► What are the goals of the chemotherapy treatment program?

► How long will the treatment take?

► What chemotherapy drugs are being prescribed?

► What are the expected side effects?

► What do you do if you have side effects?

Once you understand the reasons behind the oncologist's choice of chemotherapy, and you know what to expect, it is easier to accept some side effects knowing that the treatment is the best possible choice for your particular situation.

In the next three chapters you will learn about who benefits from chemotherapy, the different drugs and their side-effects, and typical chemotherapy schedules.

CHAPTER 31
WHO BENEFITS FROM
CHEMOTHERAPY?

Chemotherapy may be given shortly before or shortly after colorectal cancer is surgically removed, or it may be used when surgery cannot eliminate the cancer.

CHEMOTHERAPY GIVEN SHORTLY BEFORE
COLORECTAL CANCER SURGERY
(PREOPERATIVE CHEMOTHERAPY, NEOADJUVANT CHEMOTHERAPY)

Chemotherapy given just shortly before surgery is called *neoadjuvant chemotherapy*. Neoadjuvant chemotherapy is offered to patients with rectal cancer when staging tests show that the cancer is deeply penetrating (*locally advanced*) and might be difficult for the surgeon to remove. It is most often given in combination with radiotherapy for an even greater effect. The idea is that neoadjuvant therapy will shrink the rectal cancer so that the surgeon can remove it more easily and more completely. This translates into fewer complications during and after surgery, and a better chance for cure. There is also evidence that neoadjuvant treatment can reduce the number of cancer-containing lymph nodes, sometimes called "down-staging" the cancer. The course of treatment is four to six weeks. Radiation is given daily from Monday to Friday and 5-FU chemotherapy (see Chapter 32 for details) is given as an intravenous continuous infusion daily during the period of the radiation therapy. Neoadjuvant chemotherapy is not usually given before colon cancer surgery.

CHEMOTHERAPY GIVEN SHORTLY AFTER
COLORECTAL CANCER SURGERY
(POSTOPERATIVE CHEMOTHERAPY, ADJUVANT CHEMOTHERAPY)

Chemotherapy may be given shortly after surgery to reduce the risk of the cancer recurring (*adjuvant chemotherapy*). Under some circumstances this additional treatment can increase the chance for cure. Treatment should begin within six weeks after surgery.

In order to appropriately prescribe adjuvant chemotherapy drugs, doctors assess each patient's colorectal cancer and the likelihood of recurrence after surgery. In addition, they must take into account the patient's general state of health since some patients may be too frail to tolerate chemotherapy in addition to their surgery. Guidelines for who should get adjuvant chemotherapy are as follows:

ADJUVANT CHEMOTHERAPY SHOULD BE GIVEN WHEN THE
PATHOLOGIST IDENTIFIES CANCER IN THE LYMPH NODES

The most widely accepted indicator of the need for adjuvant chemotherapy is the presence of cancer in the lymph nodes of the removed specimen. If these are present, the risk for recurrence of the cancer is increased, and this is what the adjuvant chemotherapy is designed to deal with. Surgery alone will cure only about one-third to one-half of patients with cancerous lymph nodes because the cancer cells may have already escaped beyond the portion of tissue removed at surgery.

Unfortunately, the absence of cancer in the lymph nodes does not guarantee a cure. Approximately eight out of ten patients with normal lymph nodes will be cured by surgery. But in the other two, the cancer will recur even though the lymph nodes appeared to be normal. Obviously, the status of the lymph nodes is not the only predictor of outcome.

ADJUVANT CHEMOTHERAPY SHOULD BE CONSIDERED WHEN THERE ARE OTHER RISK FACTORS FOR CANCER RECURRENCE

The recommendation for adjuvant chemotherapy for patients with positive lymph nodes is based upon solid research data that shows it to improve survival. There are a number of other, less tested reasons why some cancer specialists might want to recommend adjuvant chemotherapy. These reasons are called *risk factors* for cancer recurrence. Many are being tested by current studies so we should know more about how important they are in the coming years. Still, some cancer specialists find them interesting enough to consider them in the decision regarding adjuvant chemotherapy. They include:

Cancer cells are found outside the bowel wall

If the pathologist sees clumps of cancer cells in the veins or lymphatic vessels of the colon or rectum (see Chapter 15), it usually means a higher risk of recurrence. In some treatment centers, adjuvant chemotherapy is given based on this finding.

Perforation of the bowel by the cancer

If the cancer grows through the bowel wall and causes it to burst open, the risk of cancer recurrence is increased since cancer cells may escape to the outside of the bowel.

High-grade cancer

Patients with high-grade cancers are at a higher risk of recurrence and may benefit from adjuvant chemotherapy.

A large cancer that blocks the bowel

Considered on its own, the size of the primary cancer is not a significant pre-dictor of recurrence, but if it is large enough to cause blockage of the bowel, the risk may be increased.

The cancer is stuck to another organ

If the cancer penetrates into an adjacent organ, the surgery usually entails en bloc resection of the two organs with the cancer (see Chapter 27). In such case, risk of recurrence is greater. So adjuvant chemotherapy may be recommended after surgery.

New markers under investigation

There are studies now underway to determine the usefulness of additional "markers" of risk for recurrence. These markers consist of certain genetic or molecular proteins in the cancer cells. Research has shown that the presence or absence of such markers may relate to the behavior of a particular cancer and that this information might be useful in predicting the risk of recurrence. If the results of these studies are favorable, we can look forward to using these markers to determine suitability for adjuvant chemotherapy in the future.

HOW DO ADJUVANT CHEMOTHERAPY RECOMMENDATIONS FOR COLON CANCER DIFFER FROM ADJUVANT CHEMOTHERAPY RECOMMENDATIONS FOR RECTAL CANCER?

In cases of colon cancer, adjuvant chemotherapy is recommended if the lymph nodes contain cancer cells, or any of the risk factors for recurrence (see above) are present. It is not usually given if the cancer fully penetrates through the bowel in the absence of cancerous lymph nodes. Adjuvant therapy of colon cancer is usually given without radiotherapy.

In treatment of rectal cancer, unlike for colon cancer, adjuvant chemothera-py is often combined with radiation therapy. Like treatment for colon cancer, adjuvant chemotherapy is given for rectal cancer if there are cancerous lymph nodes. But unlike for colon cancer, it is also given for rectal cancer if the cancer penetrates through the bowel wall even if the lymph nodes are normal. The reason is that the rectum is closely surrounded by tissues and cancer cells can more easily extend into these surrounding tissues of the pelvis, where they become embedded or they can reach the lymphatic vessels and blood vessels within the pelvis.

WHY ISN'T CHEMOTHERAPY GIVEN TO ALL COLORECTAL CANCER PATIENTS WHO UNDERGO SURGERY?

The reason that chemotherapy isn't simply given to everyone who undergoes surgery for colorectal cancer is that these are powerful medicines with side effects. While some groups of colorectal cancer patients appear to benefit and so the risk of side-effects can be justified, there are other groups who do not appear to benefit and exposing these patients to the risk of chemotherapy would not be helpful or ethical.

CHEMOTHERAPY FOR COLORECTAL CANCER THAT IS METASTATIC WHEN FIRST DISCOVERED OR THAT HAS COME BACK AFTER SURGERY

Patients who have metastatic disease when cancer is first discovered or whose cancer comes back after it was completely removed are usually considered for chemotherapy. The aim of chemotherapy in these situations is to control the disease by either reducing its size or preventing its continued growth. Current chemotherapeutic drugs or drug combinations may provide a clinical benefit to about 50% of patients with metastatic or recurrent disease. Those patients whose cancer gets smaller or whose cancer stays in check for a while will usually experience relief of their cancer symptoms (discomfort or pain) and an improved sense of well-being. This is particularly important in the case of rectal cancer recurrence in the pelvis, something that is not often treatable with surgery. In such instances, radiation combined with intravenous 5-FU may be used to shrink the tumor and relieve debilitating pelvic pain. The occasional patient receiving chemotherapy for metastatic or recurrent colorectal cancer may experience complete disappearance of all tumor for some time, but, unfortunately, it usually reappears.

Before the availability of the newer chemotherapy drugs such as irinotecan and oxaliplatin, doctors typically recommended that chemotherapy not be given to patients with metastatic or recurrent colorectal cancer if they did not have symptoms. This is because colorectal cancer can often run a prolonged course and patients may remain well for many months before the onset of symptoms in the event of a recurrence. Further, the older medications such as 5-FU produced only a slight prolongation of survival time in most patients. The new drug combinations available today are clearly more effective in advanced colorectal cancer and offer an improved survival to those patients treated. For this reason, there is now a trend toward starting chemotherapy earlier, once the recurrence is identified and before symptoms of the recurrence happen, rather than waiting for the development of symptoms.

THE ROLE OF CHEMOTHERAPY IN MANAGEMENT OF LIVER METASTASES
In some patients with liver metastases that may be too large for a surgeon to remove, the possibility of shrinking the cancer with chemotherapy to make it more easily removable is now being examined in clinical trials.

Hepatic artery infusion for liver metastases
The liver is the most common site for colorectal cancer metastases and in many patients, it is the only site of detectible metastases. If these metastases are limited to only a few places within the liver, surgery may be offered to remove the portion of the liver containing the cancer. Most often, however,

the liver metastases are too widespread within the liver to warrant surgery and chemotherapy might be considered.

The idea of delivering chemotherapy directly into the liver through the main artery to the liver (the hepatic artery) has been tested, with the hypothesis that perhaps the side effects of chemotherapy might be reduced to the rest of the body if the drugs can be delivered right to the liver. This would also permit a higher dose to be delivered to the liver, with lesser effects elsewhere.

To accomplish direct delivery of chemotherapy into the liver, a catheter must be surgically inserted into the hepatic artery and a pump must be implanted to deliver the drug. This requires an operation and considerable logistics to carry it out effectively. This approach has been shown in some studies to produce an increased rate of tumor shrinkage and a modest improvement of survival. The drug commonly used in this treatment is 5-FU, although the newer drugs are undergoing testing. Because of the complexity of this method of treatment and the demonstration of modest benefits, at best, this approach is not widely used and is considered an investigational treatment.

IF THE CEA BLOOD TEST IS RISING BUT NO RECURRENCE CAN BE FOUND, SHOULD CHEMOTHERAPY BE GIVEN?

Most patients with recurrence of their cancer will eventually also have a rise in the blood CEA (Chapter 13). In most cases, the cause for the rising CEA can be found with physical examination, ultrasound, CT scan or other tests. Occasionally, a recurrence may be signaled by a rise in the CEA without an obvious site of recurrence despite tests aimed at finding the recurrence. As the sensitivity of imaging improves, these situations may be less frequent. When the CEA increases without obviously detectable disease, the usual approach is to carefully monitor the changes in the CEA and re-do the imaging tests (ultrasound, X-rays, CT scan, etc.) at the common sites of recurrence at regular intervals, checking for the appearance of metastases. Sometimes, when the cancer becomes detectable, it may remain localized, for example, as a single area in the liver that may be operable. More often, however, it proves inoperable. A common site for this type of occult recurrence is the development of metastases coating the lining (peritoneum) of the abdominal cavity. This type of recurrence is not curable. Currently, most oncologists will not start a patient on chemotherapy if the CEA is rising but they are unable to find the source.

THE CHEMOTHERAPY DRUGS USED TO FIGHT COLORECTAL CANCER

The following six drugs are the most commonly used in fighting colorectal cancer:

FLUOROURACIL (5-FU, ADRUCIL, EFUDEX)

5-FU blocks the manufacture of thymidine, one of the four building blocks of the DNA molecule. The DNA of the cancer cell becomes damaged and the cell cannot divide. This kills the cell. 5-FU is given intravenously to colorectal cancer patients, either intermittently, or as a continuous infusion. It causes soreness of the mouth, diarrhea, and a temporary decrease in the blood counts (numbers of red cells, white cells, or platelets).

CAPECITABINE (XELODA)

Capecitabine is an oral (pill) form of 5-FU. The dose depends on your size, but sometimes it has to be lowered if there are side effects. It is taken twice daily, once in the morning and once in the evening. It should be taken with a glass of water within 30 minutes after a meal. The pills should be taken at the same time each day. They are usually given for 14 days, then no pills for seven days. The cycle is repeated every three weeks if you do not have any problems. It has the same side effects as 5-FU, but is more likely to cause soreness of the mouth and reddening and tenderness of the palms and soles.

RALTITREXED (TOMUDEX)

Raltitrexed is another drug that blocks the manufacture of thymidine. It is given as an injection in a vein over 15 minutes, usually once every three weeks. The dose depends on your weight and how well your kidneys are working. It causes a temporary decrease in the blood counts. Raltitrexed may also cause soreness of the mouth, but does so less frequently than 5-FU. Many patients taking raltitrexed experience generalized fatigue. It may also cause diarrhea that can become severe. It is important to call your doctor or nurse if the diarrhea does not go away in 24 hours.

LEUCOVORIN (FOLINIC ACID, FA, CITROVORUM, WELLCOVORIN)

Folinic acid is a derivative of the vitamin folic acid. By itself it is not an anti-cancer drug, but it enhances the action of 5-FU. Leucovorin is given intravenously or orally. Leucovorin has very few side effects but it may make anti-seizure medications less effective. So make sure your doctor knows if you are taking anti-seizure medications.

IRINOTECAN (CAMPTOSAR, CPT-11, CAMPTOTHECAN-11)

Irinotecan is a derivative of camptothecin, an extract from plants. It blocks an enzyme (topoisomerase 1) in cells that is responsible for making small nicks in the DNA and then repairing them. This is necessary because the two strands of the DNA molecule must first separate when they are making new copies of themselves. Irinotecan prevents the repair of the cut strands and the DNA molecule becomes fragmented, leading to the death of the cell. Irinotecan is given by an injection in a vein over a 90-minute period once weekly for three weeks and then one week off, or once every three weeks. The dose depends on a variety of things including your size, age, liver function, your blood counts, whether you have had diarrhea side-effects, and whether you have had radiation to your abdomen or pelvis. Irinotecan causes diarrhea, nausea, vomiting, hair loss, and temporary depression of the blood counts.

OXALIPLATIN (ELOXATIN)

Oxaliplatin is a new drug related to platinum. It forms cross-links between the strands of the DNA molecule and prevents the formation of new DNA. This causes the cell to die. Oxaliplatin is given as an injection in a vein over two hours. It is often given at the same time as leucovorin. It is usually followed by an injection of 5-FU, then a continuous infusion of 5-FU over 22 hours. This is repeated the next day without the oxaliplatin.

It is important not to eat ice chips or drink anything cold before, during, or after getting the oxaliplatin. The dose depends on your weight, your blood counts, and the side effects of the medicine. Its main side effects are a pins and needles sensation in the finger tips and toes as well as a discomfort in the back of the throat when swallowing cold liquids. It also causes a temporary decrease in the blood counts. Oxaliplatin can also cause a feeling in the throat like it is closing in. This sensation is scary but it does not last long. Tell your nurse right away if you get a rash, hives, swelling of your lips or tongue, or a sudden cough. You may be having an allergic reaction that can be managed.

DRUG COMBINATIONS

Different chemotherapy drugs work in different ways. To take maximum advantage of this, the drugs are often given in combinations—attacking on all fronts. Because certain combinations are used frequently, you may see them referred to as abbreviations. Some typical examples of drug combinations are:

FOLFIRI

Is a combination of folinic acid, 5-FU, and irinotecan.

FOLFOX

Is a combination of folinic acid, 5-FU, and oxaliplatin.

IFL

Is a combination of irinotecan, 5-FU, and leucovorin.

THE MAYO REGIMEN

Is a combination of folinic acid and 5-FU

Several clinical trials have examined the efficacy of these different drug combinations in advanced colorectal cancer. They have demonstrated that combinations such as FOLFIRI or FOLFOX are better than the 5-FU-folinic acid combination. A recent comparison of FOLFIRI and FOLFOX shows that the two regimens are equivalent, so patients may be offered either as the first line of treatment, with the option of switching to the other later if the first stops working.

The IFL combination was used widely in North America, but a comparison of this and FOLFOX showed that FOLFOX is better. Because of this, many clinicians now recommend either FOLFOX or FOLFIRI for advanced colorectal cancer. Oncologists continue to test different combinations of these and newer drugs in clinical trials. When a combination of drugs is given, they are usually given intravenously. Patients who are frail and cannot tolerate a combination program of intravenous drugs are sometimes given the oral form of 5-FU, capecitabine, alone.

SIDE EFFECTS OF CHEMOTHERAPY DRUGS

All drugs, even antibiotics or headache tablets, have potential side effects. What counts is that the beneficial effects of a drug outweigh the problems or discomforts of its side effects. Knowing that a particular drug or combination of drugs can effectively destroy cancer cells gives most patients the will to accept the side effects, especially if they are temporary.

It is important to be aware of possible side effects *before* you begin treatment and to discuss them with your doctor. This will make the chemotherapy process less mysterious and frightening, and allow you to decide for yourself whether the benefits warrant the side effects.

Although a number of side effects are predictable, others are not. For example, some chemotherapy drugs always cause hair loss while other drugs only sometimes affect the hair. Different people can also have different reactions to the same drug. In the last few years a number of drugs have become available which have decreased the most feared side effects—nausea and vomiting.

HAIR LOSS

Losing your hair is often the most difficult part of chemotherapy. At the doses used, some of the drugs (such as irinotecan) cause baldness for most patients. Other drugs (such as 5-FU) may cause thinning of the hair, but complete baldness is unusual.

Hair loss occurs because the chemotherapy slows down the rapidly dividing cells of the roots of the hair. Thinning usually begins about two weeks after the first dose of chemotherapy. You will notice that you are shedding in the shower, on your brush, and on your pillow. The hair breaks at or near the skin, so the scalp may be tender. The chemotherapy may also cause thinning of the hair on the rest of your body, including your eyebrows, eyelashes, arms, legs and pubic hair, but this is unusual. The hair always grows back, sometimes even during the chemotherapy. It is usually already a few inches long by the third month following completion of the chemotherapy program.

If you are to receive a chemotherapy drug that has an effect on hair, purchase a wig before you start the chemotherapy and take it to your hairdresser to get it styled so you are prepared. You can also wear hats, turbans, and scarves.

Although there have been attempts to decrease hair loss by scalp hypothermia (cold packs on the scalp) or electrical stimulation of the scalp, these are generally uncomfortable and ineffective. Furthermore, many doctors are concerned that as the cold decreases blood flow to the area, there could also be a decrease in the chemotherapy delivered to that spot, possibly leaving a potential cancer site untreated.

INFECTION

White blood cells in the blood stream protect the body from infection. After each injection, many chemotherapy drugs reduce the white blood cell count. If the white blood cell count drops too low, your body's defense mechanisms become impaired and you have a higher risk of getting an infection.

How can you protect yourself from infections while getting chemotherapy? You don't need to become a hermit but you should take precautions: avoid crowds and people with contagious diseases such as chickenpox. Wash your hands frequently and practice good skin care with frequent showers or baths. Use a soft toothbrush to avoid injuring your gums, an electric shaver rather than a razor, pay careful attention to hemorrhoids, and be on the alert for any signs of an infection. If you get a fever, sweats, chills, a cough with yellow sputum, burning urine, a sore that will not heal, or diarrhea, you should call your doctor immediately so antibiotics can be prescribed. It is rare that you would need to be hospitalized, but oral antibiotics may be required for about five to seven days until your white blood cells recover.

The white blood cell count usually recovers at about two or three weeks after chemotherapy, which is why most courses of chemotherapy are given in sessions separated by two- or three-week holidays. If your white blood cell count hasn't recovered enough to make it safe to give another dose of chemotherapy according to the schedule, then treatment will be delayed or the doses will be reduced.

A hormone called granulocyte colony stimulating factor (G-CSF for short, brand names Neupogen, Filgrastim) may be prescribed if you have problems with infection or a very low white blood cell count. This is a synthetic form of a natural hormone that helps your bone marrow recover and increases your white blood cell count after it has been lowered with chemotherapy. G-CSF is given as an injection either by the patient or a nurse every day for three to 10 days.

ANEMIA

Anemia is a reduction in the concentration of red blood cells in the blood. The concentration of red blood cells in the blood may be reduced by chemotherapy, but it does not usually drop too much.

Anemia may cause you to feel tired, dizzy, short of breath, or chilly, so if you notice any of these symptoms you should report them to your doctor. Although you should eat well, anemia caused by chemotherapy is not usually helped by taking iron or B vitamins since the low red cell count is not caused by nutritional deficiencies or bleeding but by a decreased production of red cells. If your anemia becomes severe enough to cause symptoms, your doctor may recommend a blood transfusion or an injection of a hormone called *erythropoeitin* (brand names Epo, Epogen) which may help stimulate your bone marrow to make more red blood cells.

ABNORMAL BLEEDING OR BRUISING

Platelets are elements within the blood that help it clot effectively. Chemotherapy may cause a temporary decrease of the platelet count. If this is severe enough, you may bleed easily. It is rare for low platelet counts to be a significant problem, but if you notice any abnormal bleeding or bruising you should report it to your doctor. ASA (Aspirin) or ASA-like drugs can further impair clotting by making the remaining platelets less effective. Check with your doctor before taking these medications. Acetaminophen (Tylenol) does not affect platelet function and so is generally safe if taken in moderation.

NAUSEA AND VOMITING

Most chemotherapy drugs can cause nausea and vomiting. Some people are affected more than others. Antiemetic drugs, which prevent nausea and vomiting, are usually given before the chemotherapy and every few hours afterward for the first 24 to 48 hours. Nausea may start six to eight hours after the chemotherapy injection, or even the next day, and is usually not a prolonged problem. Eat something before the chemotherapy and regularly thereafter because it is often better not to have an empty stomach.

The nausea may be worse in the morning, so it is sometimes helpful to take an antiemetic, have something to eat (for instance some dry crackers) and stay in bed for an hour to prevent vomiting. Avoid odors that cause more nausea. If the drugs you are given are not effective, tell your doctor so that different or additional antiemetics can be tried.

The drugs used to prevent nausea and vomiting include ondansetron (Zofran), prochlorperazine (Stemetil), dimenhydrinate (Gravol), metoclopramide (Maxeran), Nabilone (Cesamet), and dexamethasone (Decadron). Diphenhydramine (Benadryl) and lorazepam (Ativan) may also be helpful. Note that these drugs may also have side effects. For example, ondansetron may cause headaches and constipation and prochlorperazine may cause restlessness that may require yet another drug, diphenhydramine, for relief. The drugs may be given as pills, intravenous or intramuscular medications, or rectal suppositories. The suppositories may be the easiest to take if you are very nauseated or vomiting.

Some people also complain about stomach pain, an acidy feeling, heartburn, and a change in the taste in their mouth while on chemotherapy. These symptoms may be eased by food or antacids, but if the symptoms are severe, particularly the pain, you should notify your doctor.

Marijuana use during chemotherapy

Marijuana is known to have some value in reducing nausea and vomiting in patients undergoing chemotherapy. It is thought that the active ingredient is THC (tetra hydro cannabinol). Early studies compared THC to the best treatments of the day and found its antivomiting properties were equal to or better than oral metoclopramide and prochlorperazine, the conventional drugs most often prescribed at the time. However, there are no studies comparing THC to some of the newer drug treatments, such as a combination of ondansetron and dexamethasone. Consequently, clinicians usually consider marijuana and its synthetic derivatives to be a second or third line antiemetic therapy with a fairly uncommon role for delayed nausea and for patients who don't seem to respond to anything else.

In Canada, patients can obtain a Health Canada permit to use marijuana for medicinal purposes with the signature of a specialist, but some Canadian medical associations are advising physicians not to prescribe it. The process takes about two weeks. Unfortunately, Health Canada does not supply marijuana, and patients are expected to grow their own, which is impractical for most patients. Alternatively, they may designate an individual to grow it for them. That individual must be registered with Health Canada. There are also some compassion clubs in Canada that can provide marijuana. They are listed in the phone books of some larger Canadian cities. Compassion clubs will request a diagnosis signed by a physician to circumvent the issue of prescribing.

More information on the Health Canada marijuana program can be obtained at:

www.hc-sc.gc.ca/english/protection/marijuana.html

If you don't have access to a computer or don't know how to use the Internet, all public libraries have free Internet access and librarians who can teach you how to use it.

DIARRHEA

Chemotherapy drugs, especially irinotecan, 5-FU, and raltitrexed, often cause some change in your bowel habits, so don't be alarmed by minor disruptions. If you have cramps or severe diarrhea for more than 24 hours you should call your doctor because an antidiarrheal drug may stop the problem. A stool culture may be necessary to ensure that you do not have an infection. If you have diarrhea, try to drink lots of clear liquids to replace the fluid that you have lost and to rest your bowels. Avoid foods such as cabbage, beans, bran, and spicy foods, all of which can cause loose bowels, gas, and cramps. Milk products may also contribute to diarrhea.

Irinotecan, which is a common drug used to treat colorectal cancer patients, can cause severe diarrhea. Your oncologist, pharmacist, and nurse will give you detailed information about this. The diarrhea comes on within five to 10 days of receiving chemotherapy and is usually controllable with loperamide (Imodium). The dose of loperamide prescribed for chemotherapy-induced diarrhea is more than is usually recommended on the package, so it is important to follow the instructions provided by your caregiver. If the diarrhea persists despite loperamide, your oncologist may recommend other measures, such as intravenous fluids or antibiotics. Octreotide is a useful drug in these situations. This is given by injection three times a day for a few days until the diarrhea subsides.

Occasionally, irinotecan can cause diarrhea within hours after the drug is given. This is usually accompanied by abdominal cramps, sweating, tearing of the eyes, or light-headedness. This is treated by a drug called atropine, given either intravenously or by injection. Patients who develop this reaction to irinotecan should be given atropine before any subsequent injections of irinotecan to prevent its occurrence.

DAMAGE TO NERVES

Oxaliplatin can cause a tingling sensation in the fingers and toes due to interference with nerve function. This is aggravated by exposure to cold and tends to get worse as treatment with oxaliplatin continues. It may lead to some impairment of fine motor function, such as buttoning clothing. When the drug is stopped, the side effect slowly recedes. Also, many patients receiving oxaliplatin experience an uncomfortable sensation in the mouth and throat when they drink cold beverages, which can last several minutes. This occurs within hours of receiving oxaliplatin and subsides within hours or days. A rare side effect is the sensation of shortness of breath and difficulty swallowing coming on soon after taking oxaliplatin. It is harmless and disappears on its own, but it can be alarming when it occurs.

SORE MOUTH (MUCOSITIS)

Many of the chemotherapy drugs cause soreness or dryness of the mouth and throat. This generally appears five days after treatment begins. If this is a problem, avoid foods that irritate your mouth such as acidic, spicy, or rough foods. Rinse your mouth often with warm salt water. If your mouth gets so sore that you cannot eat, notify your doctor, as there are mouthwashes and painkillers that may ease your discomfort. People who tend to get cold sores (herpes) in addition to other mouth sores can be helped by an antiviral medication. If a white, cakey covering develops in your mouth you may have a yeast infection, which may cause mouth soreness and difficulty eating and swallowing. A special mouthwash or pill may help.

CHANGE OF SEX DRIVE

Chemotherapy drugs generally do not affect the ability to have sex, although some patients may notice changes. Some women may find the mucosal lining of the vagina becomes dry or sore and it may be helpful to use a vaginal lubricant such as Replens in such cases. As well, women may be at risk of getting a yeast infection, which may irritate the area and may require treatment with antifungal creams. Your libido, or sexual desire, may be affected by the stress of the illness and treatment, fatigue, and your anxiety about your condition. These are normal responses that are generally temporary. If you have continued difficulties with your sexual interest or activity, you and your partner may want to discuss strategies to rekindle your sexuality with a professional counselor.

GENERAL SYMPTOMS

All of the chemotherapy drugs may cause skin changes such as dryness, spots, increased sun sensitivity, or rashes. If you are going out in the sun, wear protective clothing, including a sun hat. Many patients complain about dry, gritty eyes which can be eased by eye drops or artificial tears. Other patients complain of a flu-like feeling or of feeling cold for one to three days after the chemotherapy starts.

Some patients develop joint or muscle aches and pains. These often begin after the chemotherapy is finished and can last several months. Fortunately, they are usually temporary and can be relieved with exercise or anti-inflammatory medications.

Other patients complain of "chemo brain"—a perceived loss in their short-term memory. This is usually temporary. The studies that have confirmed this memory loss have been done during or shortly after treatment. It is difficult to know if the memory loss is due to the chemotherapy, the stress of the illness, or all the anti-nausea and other medications that are being prescribed. It is also not known if there are any long-term effects (more than two years) or how many patients may be significantly affected.

Other rare side effects may also occur, so if you experience a new problem that is unexpected, even after chemotherapy is finished, you should report it to your doctor, as it may or may not be related to the chemotherapy.

PREGNANCY ISSUES

Women in the child-bearing years must prevent pregnancy during chemotherapy because these drugs, especially during the first three months of pregnancy, may cause damage and deformity to the fetus. Taking chemotherapy does not necessarily prevent pregnancy. While on chemotherapy, it is important to continue to use birth control measures; these should be discussed with your doctor.

If you continue to have periods and ovulate after chemotherapy, you may be able to get pregnant, but you should wait until you are fully recovered from the treatment and until you and your oncologist have discussed the risk of the cancer coming back. Pregnancy itself will not cause the cancer to come back, but the unpredictable nature of cancer and its potential for recurrence needs to be considered prior to a pregnancy.

If you are pregnant when you are diagnosed with colorectal cancer, chemotherapy may be given if you are in your second or third trimester and if it is important to begin treatment right away. Authors of studies have suggested that some chemotherapy drugs may be used safely during pregnancy, but this route is taken only when there are no other options.

OTHER CONSIDERATIONS WHILE TAKING CHEMOTHERAPY

While you are on chemotherapy you can eat whatever you like. However, if you are taking some other medication for another condition, your doctor should verify that it may be continued. Although some physicians and nutritionists recommend total abstinence from alcohol, an occasional glass of wine or beer is usually acceptable, but check with your doctor.

Fatigue levels vary. Some patients are able to continue their normal activities and continue working throughout the chemotherapy. Others find the chemotherapy so physically or emotionally draining, they need to take a leave from work. Although it is recommended that you remain as active as you can while on chemotherapy, you will need some extra rest. Since it's hard to predict how much rest you will need, it may be worthwhile to sit down with your family or your employer and warn them that there may be low-energy days. Also, if your job involves exposure to large numbers of people, continuing work may not be the best idea as the risk of developing common infections (such as flu) would be increased.

Physical activity is important. If you exercise regularly you may want to continue, but tone down your routine to avoid straining yourself. For example, if you run regularly, you could consider walking instead.

CHAPTER 33
CHEMOTHERAPY TREATMENT SCHEDULES

The type and duration of chemotherapy varies according to the stage of the cancer, the goal of treatment, the wishes of the patient, and his or her ability to tolerate treatment. Below are some examples of chemotherapy schedules that are used for fighting colorectal cancer grouped according to cancer stage (see Chapter 15).

RECTAL CANCER

STAGE 0: TIS, N0, M0: The cancer is in the earliest stage. It has not grown beyond the inner layer (mucosa) of the bowel. This stage is also known as carcinoma in situ or intramucosal carcinoma. This is usually a polyp. Treatment consists of removal of the polyp only. No radiation or chemotherapy before or after treatment.

STAGE I: T1 OR T2, N0, M0: The cancer has grown deeper into the bowel wall but not through it. It has not spread into the nearby lymph nodes and there are no metastases to distant sites. No radiation or chemotherapy before or after treatment.

STAGE IIA: T3, N0, M0: The cancer has grown through the bowel wall but it is still contained by the outermost layers, serosa, or mesorectal fascia, and has not yet spread to the lymph nodes and there are no metastases to distant sites. Radiation and chemotherapy are usually given. This may be before (neoadjuvant) or after (adjuvant) therapy.

Neoadjuvant therapy: To be given in one of two schedules:

> *Short course radiation* given over five days. Surgery is performed within one week afterwards.

> *Long course radiation* given over five weeks. Infusional 5-FU is also given during this period through an indwelling intravenous catheter over 24 hours per day for the duration of radiation. Surgery is performed eight weeks after the end of radiation. The reason for the delay in surgery after long course radiation is to permit the acute radiation reaction to subside.

Adjuvant therapy: Radiation and chemotherapy may be given after surgery if they have not already been used. There are a variety of schedules. Radiation will usually be given over a five week period. Chemotherapy typically consists of folinic acid and 5-FU. Two five-day cycles of 5-FU are given as intravenous injections before radiation. Each cycle consists of five daily injections of folinic acid and 5-FU. Two more cycles are given during the first and final weeks of radiation. Following this, two more five-day cycles are given monthly. An alternative to this is to give 5-FU as a continuous infusion intravenously during the radiation treatment. This is similar to that described above for long course preoperative radiation, with 5-FU given over 24 hours daily for five weeks.

STAGE IIB: T4, N0, M0: The cancer has grown through the bowel wall and the outermost layers including mesorectal fascia and into nearby tissues or organs. It has not yet spread to the lymph nodes and there are no metastases to distant sites. Radiation and chemotherapy are usually given before surgery in an attempt to reduce the size of the tumor and render it removable by the surgeon. The radiation is given over five weeks and is combined with infusional 5-FU chemotherapy given over 24 hours per day during the course of radiation. About four to six weeks after surgery, four additional cycles of chemotherapy are given. Each cycle consists of five daily injections of folinic acid and 5-FU. This is repeated every four weeks.

STAGE IIIA: T1 OR T2, N1, M0: The cancer has grown deeper into the bowel wall but not through it. It has spread to one to three nearby lymph nodes but there are no metastases to distant sites. Radiation and chemotherapy are given. The schedules are as described for Stage IIA rectal cancer.

STAGE IIIB: T3 OR T4, N1, M0: The cancer has grown through the bowel wall and the outermost layers including mesorectal fascia and into nearby tissues or organs. It has spread to one to three nearby lymph nodes but there are no metastases to distant sites. Radiation and chemotherapy are given. For T3 cancers, this is similar to the schedules described for Stage IIA rectal cancer. If it is anticipated that the cancer is going to be difficult to remove because staging tests show that it may be penetrating into adjacent tissues or organs in the pelvis, long course radiation with 5-FU chemotherapy is given before surgery. This makes it more easily removable. Once it is removed, four more cycles of chemotherapy with folinic acid/5-FU are given four to six weeks after surgery. Each cycle consists of five injections of folinic acid and 5-FU on five successive days. Each cycle is repeated every four weeks for a total of four cycles. If the cancer is not removable even after radiation and chemotherapy, then additional chemotherapy may be given with 5-FU alone or in combination with irinotecan or oxaliplatin. Another option is oral capecitabine with or without irinotecan or oxaliplatin. The chemotherapy is usually continued as long as there is some evidence of benefit.

STAGE IIIC: ANY T, N2, M0: The cancer may be any T but has spread to four or more nearby lymph nodes and there are no metastases to distant sites. Radiation and chemotherapy are given as described for Stage IIIB rectal cancer.

STAGE IV: ANY T, ANY N, M1: The cancer can be any T, any N, but has metastasized to distant sites such as the liver, lung, peritoneum (the membrane lining the abdominal cavity), or ovary. This stage of rectal cancer is usually incurable, unless there is one or a limited number of metastases in the liver or lung that can be removed by the surgeon or destroyed by cryotherapy or radiofrequency ablation (see Chapter 27). Palliative chemotherapy is usually given to suitable patients. It includes single agents (capecitabine, folinic acid/5-FU, irinotecan) or combinations of these with either irinotecan or oxaliplatin.

COLON CANCER

Unlike in most cases of rectal cancer, the depth of penetration of colon cancer and whether there are cancerous lymph nodes associated with it can rarely be determined prior to surgery. As a result, preoperative chemotherapy for colon cancer is not common. Removal of the cancer can be accomplished with good margins of safety and local recurrent disease is uncommon. As a result, radiation therapy is not generally required.

STAGE I: T1 OR T2, N0, M0: The cancer has grown deeper into the bowel wall but not through it. It has not spread into the nearby lymph nodes and there are no metastases to distant sites. No chemotherapy is given.

STAGE IIA: T3, N0, M0: The cancer has grown through the bowel wall but it is still contained by the outermost layers, serosa, or mesorectal fascia, and has not yet spread to the lymph nodes and there are no metastases to distant sites. No chemotherapy is given.

The cancer has grown through the bowel wall and the outermost layers including mesorectal fascia and into nearby tissues or organs. It has not yet spread to the lymph nodes and there are no metastases to distant sites. Chemotherapy is not routinely given, but because this stage is higher risk than Stage IIA, it may be considered if the patient is fit enough.

STAGE IIIA: T1 OR T2, N1, M0: The cancer has grown deeper into the bowel wall but not through it. It has spread to one to three nearby lymph nodes but there are no metastases to distant sites. Chemotherapy with folinic acid/5-FU is routinely given. This consists of six cycles of chemotherapy. Each cycle consists of intravenous injections of folinic acid and 5-FU over five successive days. Each cycle is repeated every four weeks. Recently, the combination of folinic acid/5-FU and oxaliplatin (FOLFOX) has been shown in clinical trials to significantly increase the proportion of patients who do not suffer a relapse within three years of surgery. As further information becomes available, FOLFOX may become the standard regimen for use in this setting. Also, clinical trials have shown that capecitabine for six months is as effective as six cycles of folinic acid/5-FU, and it is now becoming an option for treatment.

STAGE IIIB: T3 OR T4, N1, M0: The cancer has grown through the bowel wall and the outermost layers including mesorectal fascia and into nearby tissues or organs. It has spread to one to three nearby lymph nodes but there are no metastases to distant sites. Chemotherapy is given as described above for Stage IIIA colon cancer. For T4 cancer when it is felt that the surgeon may have left some behind (narrowly excised), there is a risk for the cancer to recur at that site. In some circumstances, radiation directed to this area may be considered; this is especially true for colon cancer occurring in the cecum. The radiation treatment must be carefully planned to avoid damage to the abdominal organs, such as the small bowel or kidneys. If radiation is given, the schedule is similar to rectal cancer radiation treatment, but will be individualized according to the needs of the patient.

STAGE IIIC: ANY T, N2, M0: The cancer may be any T but has spread to four or more nearby lymph nodes and there are no metastases to distant sites. Chemotherapy is given as described above for Stage IIIB colon cancer.

STAGE IV: ANY T, ANY N, M1: The cancer can be any T, any N, but has metastasized to distant sites such as the liver, lung, peritoneum (the membrane lining the abdominal cavity), or ovary. This stage of rectal cancer is usually incurable, unless there is one or a limited number of metastases in the liver or lung that can be removed by the surgeon or destroyed by cryotherapy or radiofrequency ablation (see Chapter 27). If the metastatic cancer is removed, there is no consensus whether chemotherapy given after surgery is beneficial, and clinical trials are in progress to examine this. In the meantime, treatment is individualized as to whether chemotherapy with folinic acid/5-FU with or without irinotecan or oxaliplatin is given. For those with metastatic cancer not amenable to surgical removal, palliative chemotherapy is given as described above for Stage IV rectal cancer. Unfortunately, not all patients who receive chemotherapy for advanced colon cancer derive a benefit and after a few cycles of chemotherapy, further treatment is justified only if there is demonstrated shrinkage of the tumor and it does not cause severe side effects. When there is a favorable response to chemotherapy, it may be continued as long as there is a benefit. There is a division of opinion whether patients should remain on chemotherapy until their cancer starts to grow again or whether they should receive chemotherapy only for a set period of time, such as six months, with the option to resume it when their cancer regrows and causes symptoms. The choice of what type of chemotherapy depends on the general state of health of the patient. If they are elderly or infirm and thus more likely to have serious side effects, oral capecitabine is a suitable choice. For younger or fit patients, a combination of folinic acid/5-FU with irinotecan (FOLFIRI) or oxaliplatin (FOLFOX) is the usual first choice. If the cancer does not shrink or first shrinks then regrows, the alternative regimen can be used as second-line treatment. Recently, the new agents that target specific metabolic pathways with the tumor cells have been studied in combination with the standard chemotherapy. Two that will likely be approved in the summer of 2005 in Canada are cetuximab (Erbitux) and bevacizumab (Avastin).

CHEMOTHERAPY FOR RECURRENT COLORECTAL CANCER

When a patient develops a recurrence, the first step is to use staging tests (see Chapter 13) to determine how extensive it is. If the recurrent disease is limited, such as a single liver or lung metastasis, it may be possible for the surgeon to remove it with a cure rate of about 20% to 30%. It is unclear whether chemotherapy can improve the outcome after surgery for removal of a metastasis and clinical trials are underway to get the answer.

Often, the metastases are too numerous or large for surgical removal and other measures are needed to keep the patient comfortable. For recurrences within the pelvis, radiation is usually given as it is quite safe. It is usually combined with chemotherapy (folinic acid/5-FU). Frail or elderly patients may not tolerate the side effects of this kind of chemotherapy and would do better with capecitabine, which is a more gentle treatment. Fit, young patients are candidates for the combination regimens (FOLFIRI or FOLFOX). The newer drug regimens can prolong life and for this reason chemotherapy may be commenced even before symptoms are present. However, it is not curative treatment, so if there are side effects, it may make sense to hold off if there are no significant symptoms from the cancer. The decision to start and continue chemotherapy, and what kind of chemotherapy to use, is a joint decision between the patient and doctor—with the goal of maximizing quality of life.

THREE

**BEYOND THE INITIAL
TREATMENT PHASE**

COPING WITH CANCER 14

CHAPTER 34
LIVING WITH A DIAGNOSIS OF CANCER

This section is dedicated to the emotional effects of the diagnosis and treatment of cancer—the side of cancer that neither surgery, nor chemotherapy, nor radiation can treat. Although every cancer patient and every family member is unique, the road each must travel is well-worn by the millions of others who have come before. It is a journey marked by hope and despair, courage and fear, humor and anger, and constant uncertainty. While the body undergoes tests and treatments, the mind searches for its own way of coping.

IS THERE A RIGHT WAY TO FEEL AFTER RECEIVING A CANCER DIAGNOSIS?

Many people are concerned that the thoughts and feelings that they experience following a diagnosis of cancer are somehow abnormal or crazy and that there must be a "right" way to feel. This couldn't be further from the truth. There is no one way to feel. Reactions to the diagnosis can span the full range of human emotion: anger, anxiety, uncertainty, hopelessness, helplessness, depression, a feeling of isolation, numbness, vulnerability, relief that a diagnosis has been made, and even guilt that one has somehow contributed to the development of his or her own disease or delayed in bringing it to a doctor's attention.

It is important to realize that the initial reaction to the diagnosis will be followed by other feelings. It is an emotional process that occurs. Just as we go through a series of stages in accepting the loss of a loved one, we pass through a number of emotional levels on our way to acceptance of the diagnosis of cancer. First, there is often disbelief in the diagnosis, denial that it is true, and anger at being singled out. Finally, there is acceptance. Why we go through these stages is difficult to know. Psychologists postulate that the time required to progress from disbelief to acceptance may offer protection by creating time and space for adjustment.

"I felt shocked numb like it wasn't real. I don't think I really felt anything for a week and then I felt betrayed."

"I decided that the doctors had made a mistake and that any minute someone would come out and say it had all been an unfortunate mistake."

Expressions of very strong emotion are to be expected, and they may range from anger and bitterness to frank hostility directed at anyone and anything.

"I was angry at everyone … God in particular … I hadn't done anything to deserve this."

"I just wish that they had let me die. They should just have let me go to sleep and never wake up after the operation."

As the initial anger and anxiety begin to settle, denial becomes the prominent response. Denial is a defense against fear and early on helps to maintain emotional equilibrium. You may believe that the diagnosis is wrong, that is doesn't have anything to do with you. It is not uncommon to hear people comment, "I think she's in denial," as if there may be something unusual and potentially dangerous about this reaction. In fact, some degree of denial is normal, and it is probably necessary self-protection that helps maintain the hope needed to participate in daily life. However, denial is healthy only as long as it does not interfere with seeking medical care or participating in appropriate treatment.

> "At some level I had to distance myself from the reality of the cancer in order to listen to the information that I was being given. I had to think that this was about someone else. It really protected me but it drove my husband crazy."

Fortunately, most people will emerge from the storm of emotions to reach a point of equilibrium and acceptance, although transient periods of regression are common. No one can predict when acceptance will come, as everyone is different.

> "The cancer made me realize how precious life is. I used to waste time … now I use every minute."

> "Cancer … a rare opportunity … I discovered how special my sister was."

UNDERSTANDING YOUR FEELINGS

Trying to understand the thoughts that trigger certain feelings is useful. During times of crisis, we often become more introspective. This introspection not only makes us feel less helpless but it can lead to the personal growth that many cancer patients talk about after their treatment is completed. All feelings are valid, but learning to recognize the cause of your feelings can help separate the productive ones from the nonproductive ones.

COPING WITH CANCER

Every person has a unique tool-box of coping strategies that have been accumulated over a lifetime. Most will find what they need to meet the challenge of cancer.

"How did I cope initially? I don't know, really ... I guess I did the things that I've done in other tough situations ... I turned to my family and friends, then to the nurses and doctors."

There are as many coping styles as there are people. Seeking information, turning to family and friends for support, developing a partnership with the health care team, maintaining hope, and learning stress management techniques are all ways to develop the coping mindset.

SEEKING INFORMATION

Appropriate information can help allay much of the anxiety and fear associated with the unknown. The type and amount required varies with the desires and needs of the individual and family. Generally, people want to know about diagnostic tests, the treatment plan (its purpose, expected results, side effects, length of time, and scheduling), and their prognosis. Essential but often neglected information concerns how the disease and treatment is likely to affect your daily life. Your local chapter of the Cancer Society is an excellent place to look for this kind of help. Most local chapters of the Society provide booklets, seminars, stress management training, and self-help groups for individuals with cancer and their families.

"I hated that anxious feeling; I wanted to have some control over the helplessness I was experiencing. I achieved that and calmed my panic by researching everything I could on colon cancer."

Of course, your doctor is a critical provider of information pertinent to your particular problem. When seeing your physician or other members of the health care team, don't be afraid to ask questions. They will be expecting it. Prepare a list; otherwise you may forget important points that you have been wondering about. Write down the answers and, if you wish, take someone along to help you remember what was said. One can be distracted during the early phase of diagnosis and treatment so having an extra person to listen and clearly recall is very helpful.

TELLING OTHERS

In most cases, your family and close friends will learn sooner or later that you have cancer. It is usually best to disclose the information yourself, according to your own schedule. Confiding fears and hopes is an important part of developing the coping mindset and, in the long run, it is easier than trying to conceal these important feelings.

There are some situations in which it may be best not to tell. Family members who are too old, too young, or too emotionally fragile may have difficulty accepting or understanding the situation. However, it is quite extraordinary how most people can summon the courage to adapt to the reality of a potentially life-threatening illness, even when it involves someone whom they love very much.

Sometimes family members are the first to learn the diagnosis, and they will occasionally attempt to shield the patient from the information in what is usually a misguided attempt to protect that person from the pain of knowing. In certain instances, such as when the individual is extremely old or young, or very ill and cannot understand, this is sensible. In the vast majority of cases, however, it is better for the patient to know. Otherwise, important relationships that should be strengthened become strained and artificial as loving family members and friends try to skirt the issue and discuss only superficial matters. Worse than that, in almost all such cases, the individual finds out anyway, all too often at an inopportune and harmful moment and probably from someone who doesn't even know him or her well. Don't let this happen. Given the truth about the situation, sensitively presented, the person with cancer is permitted the opportunity to evolve naturally toward the point of acceptance, and can set his or her mind on important priorities. Everyone is owed that much.

Telling young children that their parent or sibling has cancer can be especially painful. The goal in telling children that someone in the family has cancer is to give them opportunities to ask questions about the disease and to express their feelings about it. While we all wish to shield our children from bad news, it is better that they experience pain in a way that they understand and can talk about with their parents. Coping with sorrow on their own in forms that become embellished by their imagination is far less reassuring than open discussion with their family. Moreover, if they are denied knowledge of the reason for the great disruption in the family, they may become confused and hurt and mistakenly believe that they are responsible.

SUPPORT GROUPS

In many cities there are support groups consisting of people with cancer and trained professionals who manage the sessions. The professionals provide a forum where the person with cancer can be open about his or her thoughts and feelings, and can discover that these are normal and acceptable. Other members of the group often suggest alternate ways to deal with difficult issues, ways that have helped them. Seeing others who are coping with similar situations can help you identify solutions to problems that seem overwhelming initially. In addition, membership in a formal group may help you to overcome a feeling of helplessness because you will be offering assistance to others.

"Although my family was supportive, I felt as if they couldn't possibly understand what it was like for me. I needed to talk to someone else who had cancer. That doesn't mean that you shouldn't talk to your family but it's different when you talk to another survivor. In the Living with Cancer

Group, I found that I could give something back … which was very important as it was the first time in a long time that I felt useful."

A word of caution about support groups

Participating in a support group requires an investment in time and energy
that may compete with family or other activities. You may experience unexpected emotions in some group sessions. For example, you could be upset by
the beliefs or coping mechanisms of other group members. Some groups may
not be led by appropriate individuals with reliable skills or information, and
unintended emotional consequences could result. If you feel uncomfortable
or something does not feel right about any particular group, it is best to leave
immediately and seek another group.

DEVELOPING A PARTNERSHIP WITH THE HEALTH CARE TEAM

At one time, patients and families were considered to be silent members of the
health care team, if indeed they were considered team members at all. Today,
people with cancer are encouraged to take an active role in treatment planning.

Know the players

The first step in developing a partnership with the health care team is to
know who the players are and what each one has to offer. This can be a
challenging task as, over the course of time, there are often many different
specialists involved in the care of the patient and family. It is important to
identify one team member who will serve as the leader, usually the family
doctor, the oncologist (cancer specialist) or a nurse specialist. It doesn't
matter who assumes the role as long as he or she is able to relate to you
and your family and will be there for the duration. This person should be
available at regular intervals, or when required, to listen to concerns, to
direct questions to the appropriate professionals, and to serve as a guide
and a support.

Participate in decision-making

The second important step is to participate in decision-making about treatment. Although this may seem impossible because of the overwhelming amount of information to be taken into account, a skilled physician should be able to simplify the facts so that two or three alternatives can be presented at any stage of treatment.

> "I had a life threatening illness and I was being asked whether I wanted this treatment or that treatment. I felt that my life was on the line if I made the wrong decision. I didn't know whether or not I wanted that responsibility. Then I realized that I knew me better than anyone else and that knowledge would be helpful in making a good decision."

No matter how complex your problem may seem, your specialist is expected to be able to help you through the decision-making processes by providing you with a view of the big picture, thereby simplifying decisions. Once a few of the initial choices are made based on such information, you will have some time to seek additional resources and pursue the educational process that will support you later on.

Participating in decision-making means listening to the options, identifying their advantages and disadvantages, and comparing them to your own values and aspirations and those of your family. Some patients will want to discuss all of the options, perhaps seeking a second opinion before making an informed decision with or without their families. Others might be uncomfortable making the final decision, but can still participate by clarifying their values and wishes so that the final recommendations for treatment can be tailored to their needs.

Participate in the treatment plan

The third step in developing a partnership with the health care team is to participate in the treatment plan—managing the side effects of the treatment, reporting changes in your condition, attending follow-up appointments, providing team members with feedback about how things are progressing, and using the services and supports that are available. The next chapter is devoted to this topic.

A note about changing doctors

Clearly, excellent communication between you and your doctor is critically important to your successful adaptation to diagnosis and treatment. Unfortunately, some physicians never learn to speak comfortably with their patients or families and let people down by not being there for them when tough choices have to be made. Although such physicians may appear to be abrupt, aloof, and uncaring, they are usually not. Nevertheless, if this problem creates a barrier, ask your family doctor to refer you to someone else. Remember, you almost always have a choice as to who treats you, so don't be afraid to find someone with whom you are comfortable. Keep in mind, however, that a decision to change physicians should be based on reality and not on a quest to find a doctor who will promise a cure or guarantee to relieve all your fears.

WHEN FRIENDS DON'T CALL

Lost and strained friendships are a particularly painful aspect of dealing with cancer. Friends do not call for a variety of reasons. For most, it is because they feel that they will have little to say that will help and fear that instead they might say something hurtful. Others may be afraid that they will not be able to respond appropriately to your change of appearance, or they are fearful of facing the possibility of your death and the eventuality of their own.

"I see that my friends don't know how to talk to me, and they shy away from me."

None of these reasons have anything to do with your friends' view of your worth and, in fact, some may be suffering themselves from the loss of their normal relationship with you. If you believe it is discomfort that is keeping a particular friend from visiting, you might try a phone call to dissolve the barrier. This often reassures them that you are still the same person that they liked before, and that you understand their difficulty. However, don't expect to change or enlighten everyone. We all have our own emotional capabilities and timetables, and some people cannot be comforted sufficiently to enable them to maintain the relationship as it was before.

MAINTAINING HOPE

Hope is a crucial tool for people with cancer and their families. It is the internal resource that permits one to accept or better tolerate the stress associated with diagnosis and treatment. Loss of hope reduces one's ability to adjust to the situation.

Hope means different things to different people, and tends to change over time depending on the stage of the disease and treatment:

"There is always hope, it just changes. First you hope that you don't have cancer, then you hope that the cancer is curable or at least treatable. Then you hope for time and finally, you hope for a good going. If you lose hope, you give up."

Maintaining and nurturing hope is a strategy that can allay anxiety, depression, and fear. Nurturing hope means focusing on the present and what is immediately ahead, rather than on the future or the past, neither of which can be changed. While this reorientation of focus can be difficult in our future-oriented society, it can help you manage the daily challenges of cancer treatment.

Hope can be responsive to the behavior of others. Those around the individual and family must not only be aware of the hopes that are held but also should attempt to share in them or to shape them into more attainable goals.

Family members and friends can support the idea that there is nothing wrong with being hopeful and they should not classify hope as false.

> "Be prepared for the worst but hope for the best. There is no such thing as false hope. Everyday I hope for a miracle, but that doesn't stop me from continuing my treatment nor would it stop me from acceptance if my treatment is no longer working. If you took my hope away, I don't know if I would want to continue ..."

Hope is not based on false optimism or benign reassurance, but is built on the belief that better days or moments can come in spite of the situation.

STRESS MANAGEMENT TECHNIQUES

Another means of coping with a diagnosis of cancer that many people find helpful is learning stress management techniques. These are described in detail in Chapter 38.

CHAPTER 35
LIVING WITH CANCER TREATMENT

"There is more required of [patients] during treatment than just lying there and taking it: you have to report how you are doing, particularly if you aren't doing well … the information is necessary in order to help the professionals help you."

Living with cancer almost always means living with cancer treatment. While the treatment is aimed at the cancer cells, it affects the entire person, both physically and psychologically.

"How do you cope with treatment? I've had it all: surgery, chemotherapy, and radiotherapy. You either let the treatment control you or you control the treatment. It's better if you can do the controlling. You have to find out what the treatment will do for you, what side effects you might experience, and why these happen. And most important, find out what you can do to prevent or control the effects. Then you fit all of this into the other living things that you do daily. That's how you cope."

In this chapter we will discuss common side effects of cancer treatment and look at self-care measures that you can use to deal with them. Remember that you may have none of the possible side effects, or you may have several.

SKIN REACTIONS

Some chemotherapy drugs may cause the skin to become pigmented (darker), most often on the hands and feet. The pigmentation is usually permanent, although it may fade and become less noticeable with time.

A sunburn-type of skin reaction can follow radiotherapy. It develops during the second week of treatment, and lasts for the duration of the treatment and for a few weeks afterward, occurring only on the skin directly exposed to radiation. Occasionally this can break down into moist, tender patches of skin, a condition called dermatitis. This type of skin reaction is more common in skin folds, particularly in the groin, between the legs and the buttocks, if that is where the radiation is aimed. The discomfort of skin reactions can be relieved or eliminated by the following:

- Follow the skin care instructions provided by the radiotherapist.
- Avoid soaps, powders, perfume, scented creams, or deodorants on the area of skin exposed to radiation unless specifically prescribed.
- Cleanse the radiated area with warm water only, and never rub or dry vigorously but pat gently.
- Avoid anything that can scratch or injure the irradiated skin. Do not use a razor or expose the area to the sun.
- Wear loose clothing, preferably all-cotton fabrics, over the treatment area.
- Check the skin that was in the radiation field at both the entry (where the radiation was aimed) and the exit areas (where it "came out" on the opposite side of the body). Look for skin breakdown and report any to the treatment team.

THE DIGESTIVE SYSTEM

Many cancer treatments affect the digestive system. Chemotherapy and radio-therapy may cause decreased appetite, nausea, vomiting, and mouth sores. Some of these unpleasant symptoms can be prevented or controlled.

DECREASED APPETITE

Anorexia, or decreased appetite, is usually only temporary and goes away when the treatment is finished. While it is present, there are several strategies that can help:

- Eat small, frequent meals (six or more), even if you are not hungry. The meals should consist of high calorie, high protein foods that you find easy to tolerate.
- Engage in mild exercise a half-hour before eating.
- Eat when you are hungry even if it is not mealtime.
- Add dietary supplements as recommended by the doctor, nurse, or dietician.
- Consult a dietician to assist with meal planning, and contact your local chapter of the Cancer Society for nutrition guidelines for people with cancer.

NAUSEA AND VOMITING

Nausea and vomiting are among the most distressing and the most feared side effects of radiation and chemotherapy. Radiation therapy directed to the head or the abdominal and pelvic areas may lead to this. The symptoms usually begin shortly after the treatment, last a few hours, and then disappear. Some, chemotherapy drugs also cause nausea and vomiting within six to 24 hours after treatment.

For some people, the mere thought of treatment will bring on nausea. This is called *anticipatory nausea*. It is a common, psychological response and usually doesn't occur until after several treatments. The cause is anxiety about the treatment and the expectation of being ill afterward.

Both chemotherapy and radiation-induced nausea and vomiting respond well to antiemetic (antinausea) drugs. Antiemetics are taken before each treatment and at regular intervals afterward for as long as nausea and vomiting are a problem. Sometimes they can be given intravenously at the same time as the chemotherapy.

Antiemetics can be prescribed as pills, suppositories, or injections. If the nausea is severe, or if there is vomiting, a suppository is probably best. There are many different types of antiemetic agents, so if the first antiemetic does not solve the problem, others singly or in combination can probably control the symptoms.

In addition the following may be useful:

- Request that treatments be scheduled late in the day if possible. This way you will have time to eat adequately before any symptoms. Some people actually find that they have fewer symptoms if the treatments are scheduled later in the day. Of course, there are some who find exactly the opposite.
- Consider having only a light meal before the treatment.
- Don't eat favorite, nutritious foods just before a treatment so that their taste will not become associated with the unpleasantness of the treatment.
- Stick to fluids for several hours after the treatment.
- Drink at least one hour before or after eating and avoid liquids at mealtime.
- Avoid hot foods and foods with strong odors because they can aggravate nausea. This is also true of greasy foods.
- Try Sea Bands, which use the principles of acupressure to control treatment-induced nausea. The bands are worn on the wrists and exert mild pressure over an acupressure point. They come with detailed application instructions and can be purchased in many pharmacies without a prescription.

▸ Consider using relaxation, distraction, self-hypnosis, and guided imagery techniques to manage the stress of treatment. Keeping track of the patterns of both the symptoms and what relieves them will result in a personalized system of prevention—a case of being forearmed.

MOUTH SORES

Some chemotherapy drugs may lead to mouth sores that can cause pain during chewing and swallowing and therefore interfere with maintaining an adequate diet. The sores usually take several days to develop, and most are temporary. Ask your oncologist if your chemotherapy puts you at risk for mouth sores. If so:

▸ Check your mouth twice a day. If you spot any redness or if pain or sores develop, inform the treatment team.

▸ After each meal and before bedtime brush your teeth gently with a soft toothbrush, then floss. Follow this with a rinse of salt water (one teaspoon of salt to one cup of warm water). Even if you don't feel up to eating three meals a day, brush, floss, and rinse every four hours while awake.

▸ Avoid all commercial mouthwashes: they usually contain alcohol, which can irritate the lining of the mouth.

▸ Visit your dentist and dental hygienist to inform them about the treatment that is planned for you.

If you have a sore mouth, include the following in your routine:

▸ Rinse and gargle with a mouthwash suggested by the treatment team. Special mouthwashes may contain agents that relieve pain, prevent infection, and promote healing. To make eating more comfortable, use the mouthwash 15 to 20 minutes before a meal.

▸ Don't use a toothbrush or floss if your gums are sore and bleeding. Instead, rinse the mouth frequently with warm saltwater, particularly after meals.

- Avoid extremely hot, cold, or spicy foods because they can be irritating.
- Take a pain reliever before meals if one has been prescribed.
- Drink fluids at frequent intervals to keep the mouth moist and lubricated.
- Avoid irritants such as cigarettes, cigars, and pipes.
- Apply a water soluble lubricant (available at any pharmacy) to your lips to prevent them from becoming dry and cracked. Avoid petroleum jelly because it dries the mucus membranes of the mouth.

Inform the treatment team if these suggestions do not relieve the discomfort associated with mouth sores.

HAIR LOSS

Not all cancer treatment results in hair loss—it is more common with certain chemotherapy drugs than with others. Radiation, except to the head, does not cause significant hair loss. Depending on the drug or drugs involved in the treatment, hair loss may be partial, limited to thinning on the head, or complete (including the total loss of hair, eyebrows, pubic hair, and facial hair) as a result of damage to hair follicles. Fortunately, this kind of hair loss is not permanent. The hair begins to regrow within two to three months of treatment. It may even begin to regrow while therapy is ongoing.

One cannot underestimate the impact of hair loss on the way people feel about themselves during and after cancer treatment. Hair is an important part of the face that we present to others, and the loss of hair may serve as a constant reminder of the cancer. Feelings of anger and sadness are a normal reaction to hair loss and are neither unusual nor wrong. Many people describe feeling more distressed by hair loss than by any of the other side effects of cancer treatment. Important points to consider:

- Keep in mind that hair loss is temporary!
- Ask the treatment team whether your treatment will lead to hair loss and discuss possible strategies to minimize it.

- If hair loss is anticipated, consider buying a wig sooner rather than later.
- If you have long hair, one or two haircuts before treatment will make the change more gradual and less startling for you and your family.
- Keep the hair and scalp clean. Wash gently with a mild shampoo.
- Cover your head with attractive scarves and hats. These will help to disguise the hair loss as well as helping to keep the head warm. Remember that 35% of body heat can be lost from the head.
- Seek the advice of a hairdresser and cosmetic advisor for assistance with grooming. Some treatment centers offer group sessions on ways to cope with hair loss and skin changes.

PAIN

Pain is more often the effect of the disease on a particular organ system than a result of treatment. The pain of the disease will be relieved by the treatment, but if surgery is part of that treatment, of course there will be transient postoperative pain. Pain from chemotherapy is relatively uncommon. It may occur at the site of the intravenous injection of some of the drugs, or even at the tumor site. This is shortlived. In some circumstances, radiotherapy may cause a painful skin reaction much like sunburn as discussed earlier in this chapter under "Skin reactions."

Here are some ideas to help you manage pain:

- Discuss the cause of the pain and the strategies for treatment with the team.
- Take analgesic (pain killing) medications at the prescribed dose and frequency.
- Consider using relaxation, distraction, guided imagery, or self-hypnosis techniques to help control the pain. Group teaching of these methods may be available through your local chapter of the Cancer Society.

- ▶ Consult the treatment team if the pain continues or gets worse in spite of the medication.
- ▶ Take analgesic medications 30 minutes before if treatment normally causes pain.

BONE MARROW DEPRESSION

The bone marrow is the site of production of all blood cells: red blood cells, which contain hemoglobin and carry oxygen to the tissues; white blood cells, which fight infection; and platelets, which are important in clotting. Bone marrow cells are sensitive to the effects of chemotherapy. Injury to these cells may create a risk of anemia (fewer red blood cells—noted as low hemoglobin level), infection (from fewer white blood cells), and bleeding (fewer platelets).

The treatment team monitors bone marrow function by routinely scheduled blood tests. Blood samples are drawn before each treatment likely to have an effect on the bone marrow. If the blood counts (numbers of red blood cells, white blood cells and platelets) are below normal as a result of a previous treatment, a treatment may be postponed in order to allow the bone marrow additional time to recover.

A decrease in the white blood cell count does not usually occur until seven to 10 days following certain chemotherapy drugs, and the count usually returns to near normal between 14 to 21 days. When the white cell count is low the body is more susceptible to infection, so special precautions must be taken (as listed below). Platelet counts may drop a week or so after treatment and begin to build up again in two to three weeks. Care must be taken during the low period to prevent injury that might result in bleeding.

The following are some guidelines for dealing with bone marrow depression (low blood cell counts):

If the hemoglobin (red blood cell count) is low:

▸ Follow the doctor's recommendations about when to have blood tests done, and whether to take iron and vitamin supplements.

▸ Inform the treatment team if you experience fatigue or dizziness.

If the white blood cell count is low:

▸ Avoid people with colds, flu, cold sores, or any other infection. Consider staying away from crowded places for a while.

▸ Protect yourself from cuts and burns.

▸ Use sanitary napkins rather than tampons to reduce the risk of infection.

▸ Use an electric shaver to avoid razor nicks, and avoid cutting your finger and toenails too closely.

▸ Use deodorants instead of antiperspirants, which block sweat glands and may promote infection.

▸ Maintain good oral hygiene as described earlier in this chapter in the section on "Mouth sores."

▸ Do not have vaccinations updated without first checking with the treatment team.

▸ Report any signs of infection or a temperature of 38.5°C (101.3°F) or higher. Some of the signs of infection to look for include fever, chills, cough, sore throat, and a burning feeling when urinating.

If your platelet count is low:

▸ Carefully observe your skin for evidence of bruising.

▸ Avoid trauma or cuts to the skin and mucus membranes. If you do cut yourself, apply gentle pressure to the area until the initial bleeding has stopped—usually five minutes of pressure will be adequate.

▸ Avoid constipation or straining for bowel movements. Check for bleeding from the bladder or bowels by checking urine and bowel movements before flushing.

- Avoid blowing your nose too hard.

- Check your mouth and gums daily for bleeding.

- Do not take ASA (Aspirin) or any ASA-containing compound, since this can prolong any bleeding. Read the labels of any pain-killers to make sure that they do not contain ASA. If in doubt, check with a pharmacist.

- Avoid alcoholic beverages.

- Report any unusual or prolonged bleeding.

FATIGUE

Whether you are able to maintain your usual lifestyle will depend on the type of treatment and the treatment schedule. At certain times, it may be necessary to restrict particular activities. The treatment team should let you know if this is necessary.

Many people experience a period of fatigue following surgery. For some people this may last as long as three to six months. Fatigue is also a common side effect of chemotherapy and radiotherapy. In fact, it is the most commonly reported side effect of cancer treatment.

Chemotherapy seems to cause fatigue in two phases. The first phase may occur immediately after the administration of the drugs and last for one to four days. The second phase comes a week or two after treatment and is associated with anemia and a lowered white cell count. In general, the fatigue associated with radiation occurs throughout the period of treatment, and increases until the last week.

Fatigue is probably caused by many factors. It is possibly due to the buildup of waste products in the blood caused by the death of cancer cells after treatment. As the waste products are cleared from the body, some of the fatigue disappears. Fatigue may also result from the medications that are used to control the other side effects of treatment. For example, many of the antiemetic drugs cause drowsiness. Moreover, nausea and vomiting are tiring in themselves, particularly if they interfere with rest and sleep. Add to this the stress of appearing frequently for treatment and the natural sense of sadness that everyone in treatment often faces, and you have a potent prescription for weariness.

The following suggestions may help:

► Ask your treatment team about the pattern of fatigue that you should expect for the treatment.

► Plan activities to coincide with the time that you usually have the most energy.

► Provide for adequate rest periods throughout the day. Extra rest in the form of naps, a period of inactivity, a reduction in the usual activities of daily living, or a "time out"' period away from others can help you feel rejuvenated.

► Participate in a graded exercise program.

► Reassign tasks from which you gain minimal satisfaction but which take up a great deal of energy. Continue to participate in those activities which actually reenergize you (e.g., trade off a housekeeping chore for a period of gardening, which gives a sense of accomplishment).

► Enlist the support and cooperation of family, friends, and co-workers by explaining the nature of your fatigue pattern and requesting that they help you to find ways of conserving energy or using it wisely.

CHANGES IN SEXUAL FUNCTION

Cancer and its treatment may affect sexual function in both men and women, leading to decreased sexual desire, temporary or permanent infertility, or changes in sexual function. The effects on sexuality may be physically related to the disease or its treatment, or they may stem from feelings that you are somehow changed by it all.

DECREASED SEXUAL DESIRE

It is not uncommon for men or women to lose interest in sex during cancer treatment. After all, the need to deal with the reality of disease tends to crowd out other aspects of life for a while. Also important, however, is the fact that sexual desire is an emotional response to how we feel about others and ourselves, rather than a physiological response of hormones to physical stimuli. Our feelings about the way that we appear to others or the way that we feel about ourselves has a profound influence on perceptions of ourselves as sexual beings. Cancer often changes the way that we look at ourselves and may also affect our perception of how others see us. Perhaps the most difficult aspect of cancer treatment is that it influences our feelings about ourselves. While no book can change the way that we think about ourselves, nor influence the way others see us, the following suggestions may help deal with some of the factors leading to a loss of sexual desire:

- ▶ Discuss any concerns related to sexual relations before starting treatment and seek help or counseling if the need arises.
- ▶ Choose a member of the treatment team with whom you feel comfortable and discuss any concerns you may have about your sexuality and your feelings about it.
- ▶ Talk about your feelings with your partner before and throughout the duration of your treatment.
- ▶ Remember that if you were comfortable with sexual relations before starting therapy, you will more than likely continue to find pleasure in intimacy during your treatment, so make time for sexual expression on a regular basis.

CHANGES IN FERTILITY

For women of child-bearing age, chemotherapy can cause irregular or missed menstrual cycles. Women who are nearing menopause may start having hot flushes. For men, chemotherapy may cause reduced sperm counts resulting in temporary or permanent infertility. In such cases, men may consider sperm banking before the first treatment in order to ensure chances of fathering children afterwards. Because chemotherapy agents are able to alter a cell's genes, it is difficult to predict their effects on a developing fetus. It is therefore recommended that birth-control measures be used for the duration of therapy and for six to 12 months following treatment.

Consider the following:

▶ Discuss the short- and long-term effects of treatment on fertility with your partner and with the treatment team before treatment begins.

▶ Before commencing treatment, explore what options there are for maintaining fertility or banking sperm.

▶ Consider options to manage the side effects of treatment-related menopause (e.g., hormone replacement).

CHANGES IN SEXUAL FUNCTION

Treatment may lead to transient or permanent changes in physical function related to sex. For women, there may be a reduction of the normal lubrication of the vaginal lining leading to painful intercourse. A water-soluble lubricant (available at any pharmacy) can ease the situation. Avoid petroleum jelly or other oil-based creams, which encourage infection. Men may experience changes in erections or ejaculation as a result of injury to pelvic nerves by either radiation or surgery.

Discuss these possibilities with the treatment team before commencing treatment. Occasionally the answers may affect your choice of treatment, although one must constantly maintain firm priorities, with survival always at the top. The members of the treatment team are all properly trained and clinically experienced, so they will understand and be able to help you deal with this aspect of your treatment. Being aware that such situations may arise, and being able to discuss them with the treatment team and openly with your partner, will alleviate much of the inherent worry. Fortunately, modern medicine has developed a number of aids that can help restore sexual function should it become compromised.

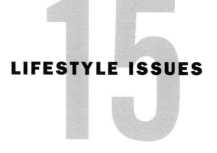

LIFESTYLE ISSUES

CHAPTER 36
QUALITY OF LIFE AFTER TREATMENT

Recovery from disease does not necessarily mean that you will experience freedom from distress. Are you free from pain? Have you been able to adapt to the unavoidable disfigurement of some of the treatments? Are you functioning psychologically, physically, and sexually as well as you did before treatment? Are you happy? These are the elements that we consider as being part of the quality of life, although no definition of the term has been generally accepted.

Not surprisingly, the notion of quality of life is difficult to measure. The literature is full of attempts to pigeon-hole patients' feelings by means of rigid questionnaires designed by investigators with no formal training in psychological assessment and who are biased by the perspective of the particular treatment they provide. For example, a young surgical resident does a research paper to determine if his mentor's patients are happy with their major surgery. Since the data is interpreted through biases and opinions, an accurate picture is elusive.

Also, patients may have their own reasons for glossing over the truth. Unwilling to hurt the feelings of their caregivers, patients often under-report their troubles. Moreover, individuals under stress have an internal adaptive process that may cause them to deny the existence of or extent of certain problems.

Suffice to say that there is a lot of bad science out there when it comes to quality of life analysis. The reality is that most physicians have little idea of the impact treatment has on patients. It has been suggested by many patients that if physicians had to undergo treatment themselves, their approach to their patients' psychological state might change dramatically.

AN ASSESSMENT OF RECTAL CANCER PATIENTS

One of the better studies in this difficult area was published in 2001 in the *British Journal of Surgery* by Camilleri-Brennan and Steele. The authors set out to assess how quality of life in patients with rectal cancer changed with time and whether certain aspects of quality of life predicted survival. Quality of life questionnaires were administered to patients before surgery for rectal cancer. Upon discharge home, and at three-month intervals after the operation for up to one year, further questionnaires were completed. Sixty-five patients participated. Those patients who developed local recurrence in the pelvis were excluded from the study. (This creates some statistical inaccuracy since those patients likely had a poor quality of life following recurrence.) The questionnaire looked at disability related to fatigue, pain, psychological and physical functioning, sexuality, body image, as well as gastrointestinal (defecation) and stoma-related problems. Also included were details about the patients' socioeconomic situation and information regarding the location of the cancer, type of operation, and whether the patients underwent radiotherapy or chemotherapy.

The authors found that in the early postoperative assessment, upon discharge home, the scores of most quality of life variables were significantly lower than before surgery. Fortunately, by three to six months following surgery, most scores had returned to pre-surgery levels. Some areas of quality of life, however, did not return. In other words, they were not as good during the year after surgery as they were before surgery. These included sexual enjoyment, male sexual performance, and perception of body image.

Regarding quality of life related to better or worse survival, the authors found that patients with the following factors tended to have the best survival:

- ► Good preoperative physical function.
- ► Good social function.
- ► Good mental health.
- ► Good energy/vitality.

On the other hand, the authors found that patients did not survive as well if they had the following factors:

- ► Advanced age.
- ► Poor preoperative general health.
- ► Reduced appetite.
- ► Preoperative fatigue.

At one year, these issues were more significant predictors of survival rate than the tumor stage, although with additional time, the tumor stage information became more directly correlated with survival.

There was a gradual return to normal bowel function over a period of one year, with diarrhea being significantly improved at nine and 12 months. Gastrointestinal problems, such as abdominal pain and bloating, improved from the third month onward. Defecation-related problems in patients who had a high anterior resection improved significantly with time, consistent with other results reported in the literature for this group. Patients with a permanent colostomy experienced a slight improvement in stoma function with time. Sexual function and sexual involvement deteriorated in the postoperative period and the latter remained poor over the year of assessment. Male sexual problems were likewise increased. Problems urinating increased after surgery, but improved to pre-surgery levels by six months. There is some evidence that modern erection-enhancing medications may improve postoperative erection problems. This is currently under investigation.

Quality of life assessment following treatment of colorectal cancer is an area of research that needs much more study.

CHAPTER 37
NUTRITION

We eat to satisfy a complex set of needs—emotional, cultural, sensual, and of course, nutritional. Eating well, in every sense of the word, is one of the most important things that a person with cancer can do for him or herself.

WHAT IS A HEALTHY DIET?

A healthy diet includes a wide variety of foods, with an emphasis on plant-based ones such as whole grain cereals and breads, vegetables, fruit, legumes (beans), lentils, nuts, and seeds. A good diet may also include lean meat, chicken, fish, and low-fat dairy products or other high-calcium foods. It also means achieving balance, that is, eating foods that contain essential nutrients such as protein, vitamins, minerals, and fiber. The Healthy Eating Plan included at the end of this chapter is recommended as a guideline. This plan can be used by patients with a variety of food preferences, including those who eat a vegetarian diet. Vegetarians should choose legumes (beans), lentils, tofu, nuts, and seeds from the "Meat and alternatives" group, and select a variety of calcium-rich foods daily.

THE BENEFITS OF A GOOD DIET AFTER A DIAGNOSIS OF CANCER

Once you have had cancer, changing your diet may also be beneficial. Eating foods low in fat and rich in vitamins, minerals, fiber, and protective compounds found in plant foods may reduce the risk of cancer recurrence. Achieving and maintaining a healthy body weight is also important, and is more easily achieved on a plant-based diet.

A healthy diet following cancer is also important for maintaining general well-being, and for preventing and treating a variety of health conditions, such as cardiovascular disease, diabetes, osteoporosis, and obesity.

IS THERE A SPECIAL DIET TO FOLLOW DURING CANCER TREATMENT?

Your body needs to have enough of a wide variety of nutrients to aid in healing after surgery or while undergoing radiation therapy or chemotherapy. The Healthy Eating Plan at the end of this chapter can be used as a guide to select foods that will provide adequate calories, protein, vitamins, minerals, and fiber during treatment and recovery.

Treatment for cancer sometimes results in side effects that may, at times, make eating less appealing. Some patients experience nausea, vomiting, weight loss or weight gain, diarrhea or constipation, a sore mouth or throat, a change in appetite, or a change in the way food tastes. Almost all will experience fatigue. Modifications to your diet, along with a once-a-day multivitamin and mineral supplement, may be recommended if you find it difficult to eat a variety of vegetables, fruits, and whole grain foods.

IF YOU ARE HAVING CHEMOTHERAPY

During chemotherapy, nausea, a sore mouth, taste changes, and mild diarrhea may occur. Ease nausea with starchy snacks and light drinks. Nausea is best controlled by a combination of medications and certain foods. Dry, starchy foods like crackers and dry cereals, eaten often, can help minimize the empty stomach feeling that can make nausea worse. Fluids like flat ginger ale, weak tea, diluted fruit juice, or ice water are generally better tolerated than milkshakes, coffee, or very sweet juices. Keeping a thermos or large cup close by can help remind you of the importance of drinking lots of fluid during chemotherapy. If the smell of cooking food makes nausea worse, try to avoid being in the kitchen, if possible. If this is not practical, consider purchased or homemade meals that can be easily reheated.

SOOTHE MOUTH SORES

If mouth sores occur during chemotherapy, certain foods should be avoided until the sores heal. Some foods to avoid include oranges and grapefruit, salty or spicy foods, or rough foods, like toast. Many patients find cold foods like fruit, yogurt, iced milk and shakes made in a blender very soothing.

IF FOODS TASTE DIFFERENT

Some patients notice that certain foods taste different during chemotherapy. For example, meat may taste bitter or metallic. If this happens, high-protein alternatives such as eggs, milk, or tofu may make eating more enjoyable. Food cravings may also occur. Some crave comfort foods during treatment, whereas others may find that fruit and certain vegetables are most appealing.

COPING WITH DIARRHEA AND GAS

You can minimize diarrhea by limiting your intake of alcohol, strong coffee, strong tea, and cola, and by temporarily eating less high-fiber foods such as bran cereals and whole grain breads. Excess gas can be at least partially controlled by eating less gas-forming foods like legumes (beans) and vegetables from the cabbage family, such as cabbage, Brussels sprouts, and broccoli.

IF YOU ARE FEELING TIRED

Previously prepared and frozen meals, convenience foods, take-out foods, or leftovers can reduce the effort of meal preparation. If possible, you might also arrange to have some meals prepared by family or friends, or use grocery delivery or catering services. Keep in mind too, that simple meals can still be nutritious—for example, a sandwich or a bowl of cereal with milk and fruit.

WHAT ABOUT GAINING WEIGHT DURING TREATMENT?

Regardless of the type of treatment you are receiving, unwanted weight gain is common. The exact cause of unwanted weight gain is unclear, but a number of factors may cause it, including decreased physical activity, eating frequently to control nausea, eating as an antidote to boredom or stress, or because of an increased appetite or food cravings. If you have recently quit smoking, you may also notice that your weight has increased.

HOW CAN WEIGHT GAIN BE MANAGED?

It's not a good idea to try to lose weight during treatment because it puts unnecessary stress on the body and can reduce energy levels as well as delay recovery. Instead, aim to maintain your weight until treatment is complete. You can do this by eating more fruits, vegetables, and whole grains, which are low in calories. Reducing the portion size of food and limiting high-fat foods will also help to achieve or maintain a healthy weight. If frequent eating is necessary to control nausea, low-fat foods are a good choice, like low-fat crackers, cereal, and skim milk, bread and jam, and fruit. Being more physically active will also promote weight loss and has a number of other health benefits. Ask your doctor or a registered dietitian for more advice.

ARE EXTRA VITAMINS AND MINERALS HELPFUL DURING TREATMENT?

Despite the popularity and common use of vitamin and mineral supplements, it is not yet clear whether their use helps in cancer treatment. Those who support their use suggest that they may restore immune function. Although a number of nutrients are required for the immune system (including vitamins A, C, E, and B6, beta-carotene, folic acid, zinc, and iron), too much of a good thing is not necessarily better and can be harmful. For example, too much zinc actually depresses the immune system.

Another popular theory is that the antioxidant vitamins—vitamins C, and E, and beta-carotene—are required to help repair cells damaged during cancer treatment. Although foods that are rich in antioxidants—dark green and orange vegetables and a variety of fruits—are recommended as part of a healthy diet, there is not enough evidence, at present, to indicate that antioxidant supplements are safe and beneficial during cancer treatment. If you are considering using high doses of vitamin or mineral supplements during treatment, discuss this with your physician or a registered dietitian.

ONCE TREATMENT IS OVER

If you have completed your cancer treatment and haven't already made healthy changes to your diet, this is the best time to start. Eating less fat and more fruit, vegetables, and whole-grain foods can give you a sense of control and well-being and enhance your recovery. Besides a possible link to cancer risk, too much fat in the diet has also been linked to the development of heart disease and obesity. In addition, low-fat diets and those rich in fruits and vegetables are being studied regarding their possible link to the prevention of various types of cancer.

You can reduce the fat in your diet by increasing the emphasis in your meals on wholesome and naturally low-fat foods such as whole grains, legumes (beans) and lentils, fruits, and vegetables. You can also limit the amount of fat by removing visible fats on chicken or meat wherever possible, and by using low-fat cooking methods such as poaching, broiling, and baking more often than frying. In addition, use less butter, margarine, or mayonnaise on sandwiches, and use light salad dressings and extra herbs and spices to flavor food. Foods such as crackers, cookies, cakes, potato chips, ice cream, and cheese are generally high in fat. It is important to read food labels to check the amount of fat and to choose alternatives such as low-fat cheese.

MORE ADVICE ON NUTRITION

You can obtain further advice about nutrition by contacting a registered dietitian at your local chapter of the cancer society or community hospital. As well, in some cities there are nutrition hotlines staffed by qualified dietitians. Check with your local dietetic association about resources in your area.

HEALTHY EATING PLAN

In one day you should eat:

5 to 12 servings of grain products

5 to 10 servings of vegetables and fruit

2 to 4 servings of milk products

2 to 3 servings of meat and alternatives

Grain products (each is 1 serving)

► 1 slice of bread

► $1/2$ a bagel or pita bread

► $1/2$ cup (125 ml) of cooked pasta or rice

► $3/4$ cup (175 ml) of cooked cereal

► 30 g of dry cereal ($1/3$ to 1 cup, depending on the type of cereal)

Vegetables and fruit (each is 1 serving)

► 1 medium size vegetable or fruit, such as one carrot, potato, apple, orange or banana

► $1/2$ cup of vegetables or fruit, such as corn, broccoli, berries, peas, or applesauce

► 1 cup (250 ml) of salad

► $1/2$ cup (125 ml) of juice

Milk products (each is 1 serving)

► 1 cup (250 ml) of milk

► $3/4$ cup (175 g) of yogurt

► 2 ounces (50 g) of cheese

► 1 cup (250 ml) fortified soy beverage*

Meat and alternatives (each is 1 serving)

► 2 to 3 ounces (50 to 100 g) of lean meat

► $1/3$ to $2/3$ can (50 to 100 g) of tuna or salmon

► $1/2$ to 1 cup (125 to 150 ml) cooked legumes, e.g. beans, lentils, split peas

► $1/3$ cup (100 g) tofu

► 1 to 2 eggs

► 2 tablespoons (30 ml) of nut or seed butter

► 3 to 4 tablespoons (45 to 60 ml) nuts or seeds

*FORTIFIED SOY BEVERAGE CONTAINS ADDED CALCIUM, VITAMINS A AND D, RIBOFLAVIN, AND B12 AND IS AVAILABLE IN SOME AREAS.

CHAPTER 38
STRESS AND RELAXATION

WHAT IS STRESS?

Stress is woven into the fabric of life. At healthy levels it challenges us and promotes activity, but when you feel overloaded or like you have lost control, then the stress is no longer healthy. The uncertainty and fear surrounding a diagnosis of cancer can lead to a feeling of overload just when there is a great need to be in control, and it can threaten your well-being.

HOW MUCH STRESS AM I FEELING?

Stress is a subjective response that is felt and expressed differently by each person. When stress becomes too great, the mind may say that you are coping, but the body gives more accurate signals. If you recognize and acknowledge your own stress response, you can begin to deal with it better.

To assess your own response to stress, learn to scan your body while asking yourself questions. Start at the top of your head, searching for tightness between the brows and eyes. Are your lips pursed? Is your jaw clenched? Are your shoulders hunched up near your ears? Normally, we don't notice doing these things until alerted by a pounding headache or lower back pain at the end of the day caused by holding muscles too tensely. Do you feel tightness in the throat, a constriction in the chest, or a churning stomach? Are you breathing shallowly, using only the upper part of your chest? Does your heart beat quickly? Some people notice that their sleep pattern is disturbed, and others eat more than they need to because eating is comforting.

When in distress, your mind doesn't focus or function the way it usually does. You may forget your own telephone number or an important appointment. Your thoughts may be dark and repetitive, and after only an hour's sleep, you may lie awake for hours doing what has been so aptly called "awfulizing." Emotionally, you are not as steady as usual, and may find yourself in tears over something that you would normally take in stride.

To be told to relax at a time like this may seem unreasonable. However, relaxation may help you find yourself filled with a tranquil energy and a sense of control. How do you achieve this elusive feeling, especially after a recent diagnosis of cancer?

HOW CAN I REDUCE STRESS AND REGAIN A SENSE OF CONTROL?

Reading this book and gaining knowledge about cancer, is one practical way to help yourself find that sense of control. Also, finding someone to simply listen is of enormous value.

Research has shown that even 20 minutes a day of relaxation can have a beneficial effect on the body. It doesn't matter whether it is transcendental meditation or simply sitting quietly watching the birds at a feeder outside the window. Twenty minutes of steady walking or other exercise works for some people. Tai-chi and yoga also use movement to bring the body and mind into a state of harmony. Meditation, in which the mind focuses on a particular word or object, or simply focusing on the rising and falling of the breath, helps to still the chattering mind and restore a sense of equilibrium. Anything that allows the body to be at ease and the mind to quiet a little seems to bring back balance and harmony. Think of the ocean. Even when a storm is raging, deep below there is a place where the water is calm. So it is with your own self. You need to find the way down to that place deep within yourself where you are calm and in control, even in the midst of chaos.

Many people are used to being responsible for others and putting their own needs last. Giving yourself permission to take some time for yourself can be an important part of the healing process. Be your own care-giver; it is important to attend to your own needs.

THE RELAXATION RESPONSE

When you relax, you find a tranquil energy and gain a sense of control so that you can respond to situations and make conscious choices rather than just react. The ancient Chinese symbol for crisis has two components, one meaning danger, the other meaning opportunity. Gaining a sense of control gives you an opportunity to make creative choices.

You can slow your racing thoughts simply by changing your breathing, especially by breathing from the bottom of your diaphragm instead of the shallow, tight breathing from high in the chest that usually accompanies stress. Try the following: take a comfortable, deep breath, hold it to the count of four and then let it out with a sigh. Repeat this four times. Feel how your shoulders release and your facial muscles soften. When you find yourself experiencing tension, remind yourself to take a sighing breath.

Autogenics is another way to occupy the thinking mind by getting it busy with repeated words such as "My right arm is heavy, my right arm is warm." By this repetition the mind starts to convince the body that its different parts are at ease. This feeling of bodily comfort induces a sense of calm control. Another way to achieve the relaxation response is to imagine yourself in a beautiful place, perhaps in nature or a delightful room, or to relive the memory of a time of achievement and strength. This is the opposite of "awfulizing" as you use your body-mind connection to create sensations of peace and connectedness. Audiotapes can also be very helpful by coaching you through these experiences (see Additional Reading).

QUICK FIXES

Sometimes finding even 20 minutes a day for relaxing seems like a tall order. You may wish to experiment with some quick fixes that will familiarize you with the healing benefits of relaxation. Whenever you are particularly stressed you naturally do one of these quick fixes already: you sigh. You can cultivate sighing as a way toward relaxation. After three or four comfortable sighing breaths you will find that the muscles of your face are more at ease, your chest feels more open, and your shoulders are softer.

Another quick fix is to practice a quick progressive muscle relaxation every time you sit down. Let tension flow from the top of your head out through the soles of your feet. Or take a 30-second vacation and recall a beautiful place or happy, carefree time.

Increasingly, you will recognize the importance of your own role in the healing process, in partnership with your physicians and the treatments and medications offered. Learning your role can add a rich dimension to the power of the partnership.

16

FOLLOW-UP AND FURTHER TREATMENT

Follow-up refers to a program of visits to the family physician or specialist following recovery from treatment. It is necessary for two reasons: first, because the patient who has had a colorectal cancer treated is at risk of a recurrence of that cancer. A recurrence means that the same cancer grows back. Early detection of that recurrence may permit it to be cured by a second operation. Second, follow-up is needed even if the operation cured the patient because a person who has had one colorectal cancer is at risk of developing a second one in another area of the remaining colon or rectum.

THE MAGIC FIVE YEARS—AND THE CRITICAL TWO YEARS

It is uncommon for a colon or rectal cancer to recur more than five years after surgery. Accordingly, the five-year mark is used to determine if a patient is cured of the cancer. If a colon or rectal cancer is going to recur, either locally

---

*These guidelines do not necessarily apply to patients with familial adenomatous polyposis, hereditary non-polyposis colorectal cancer (HNPCC), or ulcerative colitis types of cancer.

(in the area of the original cancer) or as metastases elsewhere in the body, most often it will do so within the first two years after surgery. More than 75% of all recurrences will make themselves known during these first 24 months. Therefore, people who get through the first 24 months without evidence of recurrence have a very good chance of being cured. Because of this, follow-up routines become less rigorous as the third post-surgery year begins.

IS FOLLOW-UP WORTHWHILE?

There are those who suggest that once the full treatment for colorectal cancer has been given, follow-up is a waste of time. They argue that little can be done for most patients who develop a recurrence, so the frequent visits and tests only serve to create costs and anxiety—better the patient not know whether the cancer is returning. Moreover, some patients, through follow-up, will come to know that their cancer is re-growing and is now incurable well before they have any symptoms. This burdens them with an unnecessary and perhaps unfair knowledge that creates significant psychological stress and affects their remaining symptom-free days.

Unfortunately, it is true that the majority of patients who develop a recurrence of colon or rectal cancer cannot be cured of it, and perhaps they are put through the stress of follow-up without benefit. But there is a dilemma in that there is a small group of patients who develop a recurrence who are still curable provided that the recurrence is identified early. One never knows who they will be, so the entire group becomes burdened by the stress of follow-up in order to identify those select individuals who can be helped. Clearly this is unfair, but there seems to be no alternative at present.

The patients who stand the greatest chance of a cure after recurrence are those with recurrence at the anastomosis, in the buttock skin after abdomino-perineal operation, or as a single metastasis in the liver or lung. Cure rates of up to 25% have been reported in these patients following re-operation.

Recurrence in the pelvis outside of the rectum or elsewhere in the abdomen or lungs as multiple metastases is rarely curable.

"CLEARING" COLONOSCOPY

Ideally, colonoscopy should be performed before surgical treatment. If this did not occur, then it should be done three to six months after surgery. This is to ensure there are no other polyps or malignancies in the colon that might have been missed. A high quality barium enema combined with sigmoidoscopy is an acceptable alternative where colonoscopy is not readily available.

WHO SHOULD DO THE FOLLOW-UP?

Follow-up is best done by the surgeon who did the operation, particularly after localized procedures (see Chapter 26). In addition, there may be psychological reasons why follow-up with the surgeon is useful. The surgeon is often seen as the provider of the most definitive part of the cancer treatment, and patients see that role as the one most associated with a feeling of hopeful outcome. Although it may be somewhat irrational, patients often report a feeling of abandonment if they are not permitted to follow-up regularly with their surgeon. Some surgeons who are aware of this will often continue to see their patients through many years of follow-up until they have reached the five-year survival point, in order to provide that added psychological comfort. Nevertheless, there are some situations, such as geographic distances between the surgeon and the patient, that will dictate that follow-up be done by the family physician.

OFFICE VISITS

After the usual postoperative checks that are normally done within a few weeks of leaving hospital, the patient should be seen for cancer follow-up every three months for the first two years. Any patient problem should be discussed and a general physical examination performed. If the patient is being followed by a surgeon after anterior resection or localized treatment (see Chapter 26) for rectal cancer, the surgeon will want to examine the rectum with a sigmoidoscope. Certain cases of recurrence of cancer at the anastomosis after rectal cancer surgery are curable if the anastomosis is surgically removed.

Follow-up sigmoidoscopy is also useful in identifying healing problems at the anastomosis such as excessive narrowing, which would make bowel movements difficult.

CHECKING TUMOR MARKERS

Some colorectal cancers produce a protein called CEA which can be measured in the blood. Normally, the blood level of CEA is less than five units. For a patient suspected of having a colon or rectal cancer, a CEA level taken before surgery is useful information because it can be used to compare with CEA levels after surgery and during follow-up. If the CEA level is above normal before surgery, it should fall to within the normal range afterward, indicating that all cancer has been removed. To confirm that it has returned to normal after treatment, the CEA level should be measured a few weeks after surgery. If this postoperative level is normal but then rises to an abnormal level over a period of months or years, it is a strong indicator of recurrence of cancer. If the CEA does not go down to normal shortly after surgery, it could mean that there are unidentified metastases.

After the initial postoperative measurement, CEA should be measured every three months for the first two years, then every six months for the next three years. In the majority of cases, a rising CEA postoperatively indicates a situation that is not curable. But it is only by following the CEA that one can identify the uncommon patient whose rising CEA is a marker of a single metastasis in the liver or lung. In some reports, up to 25% of such patients have been cured by surgery that removes these single metastases.

PREVENTING NEW CANCERS

Patients who have had one colorectal cancer are at increased risk for developing another one. All colorectal cancer patients who have not developed a recurrence should have a colonoscopy once every three years until no new adenomatous polyps are found. Thereafter, a colonoscopy every five years is recommended. A high quality barium enema combined with sigmoidoscopy is an acceptable alternative where colonoscopy is not readily available.

WHERE CAN DISEASE RECUR?

Overall, colorectal cancer will recur in about 50% of patients who have been treated for cure. The likelihood of recurrence will vary with the stage and the grade of the cancer (see Chapter 15). A cancer can recur in its original site (local recurrence) or elsewhere in the body (by metastasis). Unfortunately, in many cases, both types of recurrence happen simultaneously. In only half of the patients who develop local recurrence will the recurrence be an isolated one. This is one of the key issues doctors take into account when treating recurrent disease. If an area of recurrent disease can be shown to be isolated, aggressive treatment is often warranted. However, if the recurrence is not isolated, the chance of cure is small and large operations may not be justifiable.

HOW IS RECURRENCE DETECTED?

In patients who have had surgery for rectal cancer, the way that a recurrence is discovered depends upon what operation was performed. In those who underwent an anterior resection and still have an anus, 80% of recurrences in the pelvis (local recurrence) are diagnosed by digital rectal exam and simple rigid sigmoidoscopy. In contrast, local recurrences after an abdominoperineal resection and colostomy cannot be diagnosed in this way since there is no longer an anus for digital examination. Local recurrence after abdominoperineal resection is usually identified by pelvic CT scan after the patient experiences pain or has an elevated CEA blood test. For these reasons, local recurrence after abdominoperineal resection tends to be identified up to 12 months later than in those who had an anterior resection.

In 40% of patients with local recurrence, the problem is identified before any symptoms arise. Of the patients who do have symptoms, over half have pain, 20% have bleeding, 10% have intestinal blockage, and the remainder have various symptoms including weakness, sensory loss, and urinary incontinence. An elevated CEA can help identify a problem, but a normal CEA does not exclude the possibility that local recurrence is taking place in the pelvis. About half of patients with a diagnosis of local recurrence will have a normal CEA. For reasons that are unclear, recurrence outside of the pelvis seems to be more likely to cause an elevated CEA than when the disease is confined to the pelvis.

LOCAL RECURRENCE OF RECTAL CANCER

Patients undergoing curative resection for rectal cancer have a 4% to 30% risk of developing local recurrence of rectal cancer. The reasons for recurrence include biologically aggressive cancer, inaccurate preoperative staging (underestimating the initial extent of tumor spread), and inadequate surgical removal.

There are many complex structures in the pelvis. Some, like the bladder, can be removed along with a recurrent cancer—with the hope of cure. Other structures are not removable, so it makes sense to classify the types of local recurrence into different groups in order to provide guidelines for treatment. The type of local pelvic recurrence dictates what type of treatment is possible.

RECURRENCE SOLELY AT THE ANASTOMOSIS

Sometimes, rectal cancer will recur right at the anastomosis, where the bowel is rejoined in an anterior resection. If it is isolated to this spot, re-operation may result in a cure in up to 40% of cases. Unfortunately, isolated anastomotic recurrence is rare, making up less than 5% of all local recurrences. In most cases, careful assessment will show that there is also adjacent additional cancer in the pelvis (often connected to the cancer that can be seen at the anastomosis), or elsewhere in the body. If the recurrence seems isolated and surgery is planned, a repeat anterior resection or abdominoperineal resection should be performed depending upon how high the anastomosis is above the anus. A repeat anterior resection may be possible if the first anastomosis is high enough. If not, an abdominoperineal operation may be proposed.

RECURRENCE FOLLOWING LOCAL EXCISION OF A SMALL RECTAL CANCER

If the initial operation was a trans-anal excision of a low rectal cancer (see Chapter 26) and follow-up identifies a recurrence within the rectal wall at the site of excision, the situation should be treated according to the guidelines for recurrence at the anastomosis noted in the preceding paragraph.

ISOLATED RECURRENCE IN THE BUTTOCK SCAR FOLLOWING ABDOMINOPERINEAL RESECTION

Another rare type of potentially curable recurrence, called *perineal recurrence*, is due to spillage of cancer cells at the time of an abdominoperineal resection (during the course of removal of the rectum from below). The cancer cells begin to grow in the buttock wound, creating a lump there. If this is the only site of recurrent cancer, excising the area can cure the patient. However, as in the case of anastomotic recurrence, patients with a perineal recurrence may have more cancer deeper in the pelvis or elsewhere.

ANTERIOR PELVIC RECURRENCE

Anterior means toward the front. A rectal cancer that recurs anteriorly in the pelvis in men may invade the prostate gland and bladder. In women it may invade the vagina, uterus, and bladder. All of these organs are removable, although with a significant physical and emotional cost to the patient. In women, the uterus separates the rectum from the bladder, so bladder invasion in women is less common than in men. In an anterior recurrence in men, the operation of removing the bladder and prostate and recurrent cancer is called a *total pelvic exenteration*. This leaves the patient with both a colostomy for stool and also a urine stoma on the abdominal wall. These operations are extreme and drastic, and should only be done in fit patients who have been rigorously studied to ensure that the disease is isolated to those areas that can be removed. In suitable patients, there have been some cases of cure.

POSTERIOR PELVIC RECURRENCE

Posterior means toward the back. Posterior pelvic recurrence of rectal cancer is recurrent cancer in the tissue behind the rectum. Behind the rectum lies the tailbone (sacrum). Posterior recurrence will usually mean that the recurrent cancer is penetrating into the sacrum. Curing this situation may be possible in some cases by removing the recurrence along with a portion of the sacrum. Removing a part of the sacrum is technically very challenging for the surgeon and is a highly specialized operation that may take four to 12 hours and will typically involve significant blood loss. The surgical team will need to include an orthopedic surgeon or spine surgeon with experience in removing the portion of sacrum involved. The chance of dying from the operation alone approaches 10%, and the complication rates are at least 50%. If part of the sacrum is removed along with anterior organs such as the bladder, the surgery is called a *composite resection* (anterior and posterior), and is an even bigger procedure.

NON-RESECTABLE PELVIC RECURRENCE

There are some types of local recurrence that should usually not be operated on because they have not been associated with cure. They include the following situations:

- ► Recurrent rectal cancer that involves the side wall of the pelvis. Operations to remove the muscles, nerves, blood vessels, and bone in these areas are extensive and dangerous and have not been found to be of benefit.
- ► Recurrent rectal cancer that involves the upper parts of the sacrum. Since the upper sacrum is required for pelvic stability and the upper sacrum contains large nerves required for control of the legs, removal of the upper sacrum is not reasonable.
- ► Recurrent rectal cancer that involves the large nerves exiting from the pelvis to the legs (sciatic nerves).
- ► Recurrent rectal cancer that blocks both ureters (the tubes that transport urine) on their course from the kidneys to the bladder. This is a sign of extensive recurrence in the pelvis.
- ► Recurrent rectal cancer that extends upward to involve the small intestine.
- ► Any recurrent rectal cancer in which there is recurrent disease also found outside of the pelvis, except in very unusual circumstances.

SURGERY FOR RECURRENT DISEASE OUTSIDE OF THE PELVIS

Colon cancer, because it was never in the pelvis, rarely recurs in the pelvis except in very advanced cases. It may recur in the abdomen close to where it lay originally, especially if it was a cancer that penetrated through the bowel wall and was present on the outside of the bowel at the time of surgery. Recurrences in such areas are difficult to treat surgically since they are usually widespread in the area by the time they are identified.

Both colon cancer and rectal cancer can recur by metastases (spreading to different parts of the body). The most common locations for colorectal cancer metastases are the liver and lungs. Unlike other cancers (such as prostate cancer), colorectal cancer rarely spreads to the bones until very late in the disease, if at all. There is a chance for cure if a colon or rectal cancer recurs as a single or very limited number of metastases (three or less and all in the same area) in the liver or lung. In cases that are carefully assessed to ensure there is no cancer in other areas, surgical removal of a solitary liver metastasis is associated with cure in up to 25% of cases. See Chapter 27 for additional information on the treatment of metastases.

WHAT MUST BE DONE BEFORE DECIDING TO GO AHEAD WITH SURGERY FOR RECURRENT COLORECTAL CANCER?

Except for the rare case of an isolated buttock scar recurrence after abdominoperineal resection (perineal recurrence), all operations for recurrent colorectal cancer are highly specialized and may involve significant risk and recovery time. Patients and their doctors must ensure that there are reasonable hopes for cure. The cancer team must be very careful to identify all possible sites of the cancer. Only half of patients with local recurrence will have isolated disease. Unfortunately, extensive pelvic surgery in those with cancer elsewhere has virtually no chance of curing the patient. Only when the surgeon is confident that the recurrence is isolated and can be removed without undue risk to the patient should he or she go ahead.

Appropriate tests to determine the stage of a colorectal recurrence include CT scan of the abdomen, pelvis, and chest, colonoscopy to ensure there are no other cancers, MRI of the pelvis, bone scan, and PET scan. Sometimes a laparoscopic assessment of the abdomen or pelvic examination of the patient under anesthetic (when the patient is entirely relaxed) can help the doctor assess abdominal metastases or the extent of involvement of tissues in the pelvis.

THE ROLE OF RADIATION AND CHEMOTHERAPY IN RECURRENT CANCER

Radiation and chemotherapy are often used in the management of recurrent cancer, depending on where the recurrent disease is and what treatment might already have been given. (See Chapters 18 and 33 for more information.)

OUTCOME OF TREATMENT FOR RECURRENT COLORECTAL CANCER

This is an area where interpreting the scientific literature is very difficult for the following reasons:

- ► Most published studies report on very few patients so they don't necessarily reflect what would happen if larger numbers of patients were included.
- ► Each patient presents different signs and symptoms given the numerous ways that colorectal cancer can recur, so grouping them together may not provide useful data when considering an individual.
- ► The patients may have had different quality of initial surgery (those who recur following an inadequately resected mesorectum for rectal cancer may respond more favorably to expert repeat surgery than those who have recurred after a well-performed mesorectal excision).
- ► The patients may have had different auxiliary treatments when they were first treated (for example, those who have had radiotherapy with their initial surgical treatment do not do as well from subsequent surgery than those who have not).
- ► The patients may have had different types of treatment for their recurrent disease.

▸ The actual results of many fine surgeons differ from written accounts describing excellent results after surgery for recurrence. Guided by their personal experience with these operations, these surgeons cannot help but be somewhat pessimistic about recurrent colorectal cancer surgery and a bit suspicious about those who report outstanding results.

As a result of all of these issues, your physician can only extrapolate cautiously from the literature when discussing your possible outcome.

In the uncommon situation in which disease is confined solely to the anastomosis, the cure rate may approach 40% to 50%. Surgery for anterior recurrence involving adjacent pelvic organs is associated with a 15% to 38% five-year survival. If the sacrum is invaded (posterior recurrence) at a level low enough to be removed (segment S3 of the sacrum or lower), surgery may yield a five-year survival in up to 10% of cases treated. In some studies, local recurrence amenable to combined anterior and posterior resection has shown a 10% to 35% five-year survival, but not many surgeons would feel confident that they could reproduce these results. As noted above, many surgeons consider these results to be unrealistically good, particularly for anterior recurrence or combined anterior/posterior recurrence.

CHAPTER 41
PALLIATIVE TREATMENT IN
COLORECTAL CANCER

Palliative treatment is treatment designed to relieve symptoms in the incurable patient. The goal of palliative treatment is to improve or maintain quality of life. Given that so many treatments reduce quality of life in the short term, palliative treatment must be thoughtfully and judiciously applied so that the patient's remaining time is not impaired by treatment complications.

THE ROLE OF SURGERY IN PALLIATIVE TREATMENT

The goals of surgery in palliative treatment are to control symptoms and prevent complications that might occur without surgery. The surgeon must determine whether symptoms will become an uncontrolled problem prior to death and whether the procedure can be accomplished without significant risk of death or complications. If the answer is yes to both of these questions, then a palliative operation can be contemplated provided the patient is aware of the potential risk and benefits. If the risks far outweigh the benefits of surgery, then non-surgical options are more sensible.

CONTROL OF SYMPTOMS

Symptoms consist primarily of pain, bleeding, and obstruction. If the patient experiences pain in the area of recurrent cancer, surgery is usually not the best treatment. Radiotherapy, if appropriate to that location, can be more effective and less risky.

Sometimes a recurrent tumor mass will grow large enough to block the bowel. This can lead to severe abdominal cramping pain because the bowel repeatedly goes into spasm as it tries to push contents past the obstruction. An operation to relieve the obstruction should be offered in order to rid the patient of the obstructive pain. The operation may involve diverting the stool into a stoma above the obstruction rather than attempting to remove the actual obstructing tumor.

Recurrent cancers do not often bleed significantly. However, in rare cases, bleeding into the bowel can become enough of a problem to require treatment. Surgery is not often used in these cases since such a recurrence is usually substantial and operating could involve significant risk. Radiotherapy may be more effective for those patients.

PREVENTING COMPLICATIONS

If a recurrent cancer is large and looks as though it could soon cause a bowel obstruction, it might be reasonable to operate ahead of time in order to divert the stool into a stoma above the level of obstruction. This could be preferable to waiting until an emergency operation for complete obstruction would be required. This is particularly important if there is a plan to provide palliative radiotherapy to a recurrent cancer mass that is beginning to block the bowel. Radiotherapy can cause such a mass to swell, and this could lead to an emergency bowel obstruction. Operating to give the patient a stoma prior to radiotherapy creates a much more controlled situation, since swelling of the mass following radiotherapy will, in this case, not cause any particular problem.

THE ROLE OF RADIOTHERAPY IN PALLIATIVE TREATMENT

Radiotherapy given to relieve symptoms from cancer that has spread and is not amenable to cure is called *palliative radiotherapy*. Palliative radiotherapy may be given to almost any site of metastases. The treatment schedule will depend on the site of disease, the patient's state of health, and his or her life expectancy. Most palliative treatment courses last between one day and two weeks. It is important to understand that the purpose of palliative radiotherapy is to relieve symptoms. It is not generally given in the absence of symptoms, so there may be situations when treatment for incurable disease is deferred or not recommended at all because that particular area of disease is not causing any symptoms and there is no potential benefit from treatment at that time.

THE ROLE OF CHEMOTHERAPY IN PALLIATIVE TREATMENT

For patients who are having symptoms from incurable recurrent disease or metastases, chemotherapy may help. Combination chemotherapy (e.g., FOLFIRI or FOLFOX; see Chapter 32 for details) may be recommended for those who are fairly fit. For elderly patients, oral chemotherapy with capecitabine may be more appropriate. As in other palliative treatment, the aim is to improve patient comfort. About half of the patients treated this way can expect some improvement in pain and sense of well being.

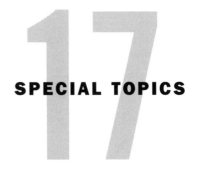

SPECIAL TOPICS

HOW COMMON IS HEREDITARY COLORECTAL CANCER?

In 75% of patients with colorectal cancer, there is no family history. These patients have what is called *sporadic colorectal cancer*. In 20% of patients with colorectal cancer there is a family history but no strong hereditary syndrome. These patients have what is called *familial colorectal cancer*. In the remaining 5% there is a family history pattern in which a hereditary association seems clear. These patients have what is called *hereditary colorectal cancer*.

CANCER AND GENES

Every one of our cells contains strands of genes called chromosomes. Genes contain the codes which the cell uses to make proteins. These proteins determine how the cell will function. All of our cells, except sperm and egg cells, contain 23 pairs of chromosomes. We have two copies of each gene, because we inherit one copy of each chromosome from each parent.

All cancers are the result of damage to genes. Most of that damage occurs during the course of our adult lifetime, which is why cancer is more common in older people. In some cases, however, a person is born with one copy of a gene that already has a problem, a *mutation* that was passed down from a parent and increases the risk of developing cancer. This is what causes hereditary cancer—an abnormal gene that is passed down in a family, a gene that carries with it an increased risk for cancer.

THE COLORECTAL CANCER GENES

In families who have a suspected *hereditary colorectal cancer* syndrome, the inheritance pattern always follows a classic distribution of genetic disease called *autosomal dominant inheritance*. This means that both males and females have a 50% chance of inheriting the gene mutation and thereby inheriting the increased cancer risk, as described in the next paragraph.

A person who inherits a colorectal cancer gene mutation is born with one normal copy of the gene and one mutation copy in every cell. Each time that person has a child, he or she can pass on either the mutation copy or the normal copy of the gene. This means that each child has a 50/50 chance of inheriting the gene mutation and the increased cancer risk that it causes. However, each child also has a 50/50 chance of inheriting the normal copy of the gene. The child who inherits the normal copy of the gene would not have an increased cancer risk and could not pass the mutation on to their children since they would not possess it in any of their cells.

THE HEREDITARY COLORECTAL CANCER SYNDROMES

Hereditary colorectal cancer has two well-described forms: *familial adenomatous polyposis* (FAP) and *hereditary non-polyposis colorectal cancer* (HNPCC).

FAMILIAL ADENOMATOUS POLYPOSIS (FAP)

Familial adenomatous polyposis (FAP) is the less common of the two hereditary colorectal cancer syndromes but it is a striking disease and the best-
understood inherited colorectal cancer syndrome.

FAP accounts for 1% of colorectal cancer cases. The main feature of FAP
is that young people develop hundreds or thousands of polyps in the colon
(Figure r, color section). By age 35, 95% of people with FAP will have *polyps.*
These polyps are adenomas, and so they have the potential to transform into
cancers (see Chapter 6 for details). It was the study of FAP that led to the
understanding that adenomas can transform into cancers (the so-called
"polyp-cancer sequence"). If the polyps are not removed, 100% of affected
patients will develop colorectal cancer by age 40. The average age of development of colorectal cancer in FAP is between ages 20 and 35. Other features
of FAP may include: polyps in the stomach or small bowel, missing or extra
teeth, lumps on the bones, cysts of the skin, and other kinds of cancer.
When these other features are present, in addition to the colon polyps, the
disease is sometimes referred to as *Gardner's syndrome.*

FAP is related to a mutation in a *tumor suppressor gene.* This gene acts
like a traffic signal, allowing specific cells to divide only at specific times. If
a tumor suppressor gene in a cell is damaged, that cell may begin to divide
without control and cancer may develop.

The tumor suppressor gene in this case is the APC (*adenomatous polyposis coli*) gene at chromosome band 5q21. It is the best known of all colorectal
cancer-associated genes.

The family tree depicted in Figure 32 shows a typical FAP family history.
The grandfather and one of his daughters died (diagonal slash) of colorectal
cancer at very young ages. Another daughter, who was found to have FAP
at age 22, had her colon removed (colectomy) and is now 59 without having
had colorectal cancer. The woman who brought the family to the attention

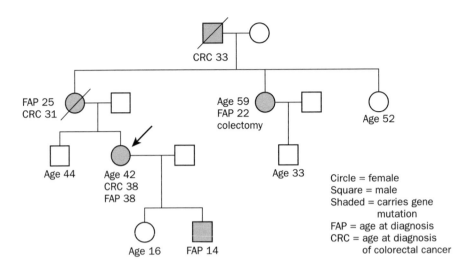

Figure 32. *A FAP family history.*

of a genetics program (arrow) has had colorectal cancer and was diagnosed with FAP at age 38. Her brother, daughter, and son have had genetic testing for FAP, with only the 14-year-old son being found to carry the FAP gene mutation. The son is being examined regularly and will likely have his colon removed before he turns 15.

The age of onset of adenomas in the colon in FAP is variable. By age 10, only 15% of FAP gene carriers have polyps; by age 20 they will be seen in 75%; by age 30, 90% will have polyps. If something is not done, 100% of FAP patients will have colon or rectal cancer by age 40. For those thought to be at risk, screening should begin very early and should consist of yearly rigid sigmoidoscopy beginning at the age of 10 to 12 continuing until age 50. Initially, a smaller instrument is used in young patients. It is best to have a supportive parent present and a very gentle and understanding examiner. Sigmoidoscopy is chosen over colonoscopy because it is less invasive and because it is thought that polyps will rarely occur elsewhere without also being present in the rectum. When the patient is a bit older, say 16 years old, flexible sigmoidoscopy, with its longer reach, may be a more appropriate screening tool.

Genetic testing for APC gene mutations is now commercially available. Depending upon the testing method used, 80% to 95% of APC gene mutations can be detected. A person whose test is negative for an APC gene mutation that has been identified in another family member does *not* have FAP and, therefore, does not have an increased risk to develop colorectal cancer. This means that screening as described above does not need to continue (or start). Some experts suggest that one flexible sigmoidoscopy or colonoscopy examination should be performed in early adulthood (by age 18 to 25) to confirm the genetic test result and the absence of FAP.

If a young, high-risk individual being screened for FAP is found to have even a couple of polyps, he or she likely has the disease and needs to be followed very carefully. If he or she continues to show the development of additional polyps, surgical removal of the entire colon with or without the rectum will eventually be required to prevent death from colorectal cancer. Timing of the colectomy should be determined by the patient and a colorectal surgeon. If the patient is still young and there are not many polyps, regular colonoscopic surveillance (every six to 12 months) may be appropriate for a few years. But when too many polyps develop, continued colonoscopic surveillance becomes inadequate and colectomy is necessary. Rectum-sparing surgery, where the colon is removed and the small intestine is reconnected to the top of the rectum (colectomy and ileorectal anastomosis), is a reasonable alternative to complete removal of both the colon and rectum, provided the patient understands the potential requirement for further surgery if too many polyps develop in the rectum. A more common surgical option now is colectomy and pelvic pouch, where the rectum is removed and the small intestine is used to construct a rectum-like reservoir (pouch) that is stapled to the top of the remaining anus.

In addition to developing colorectal cancer, patients with FAP are at increased risk for other types of malignancies including thyroid cancer, stomach and duodenal cancer, small bowel cancer, liver tumors, and brain cancer. The risk of these tumors is much lower than the risk of colon cancer, but it is recommended that the esophagus, stomach, and duodenum be examined periodically in FAP patients as polyps can develop in those areas.

Attenuated FAP (AFAP)

Attenuated FAP (AFAP) is a variation of FAP characterized by fewer than 100 polyps (30 on average). The average age that people with AFAP develop colorectal cancer is in the early 50s, later than in FAP. Its incidence is not known, though it may be just as rare as FAP. AFAP can also be associated with the other types of tumors also seen in FAP. It has been suggested that screening for people with suspected AFAP should be done by colonoscopy since it is less certain that polyps will occur in the rectum given the lesser number of polyps overall. Screening should begin at age 18 to 20. AFAP is associated with the APC gene, and genetic testing is available.

A special version of FAP within the Ashkenazi Jewish population

Another variation of FAP has been linked to one specific mutation in the APC gene, found in about 6% of people of Ashkenazi Jewish descent. This mutation (I1307K) appears to increase the lifetime risk of colon cancer but only by 10% to 20% (approximately double the risk in the general population). A person who carries this gene mutation should start to have regular colonoscopy at age 35, or five to 10 years younger than the age of the youngest colon cancer diagnosis in the family. Genetic testing for the I1307K mutation is available and provides a conclusive positive or negative test result.

HEREDITARY NON-POLYPOSIS COLORECTAL CANCER (HNPCC)

Hereditary non-polyposis colorectal cancer (HNPCC) is also called *Lynch syndrome* or *cancer family syndrome*. HNPCC is different from FAP in that people do not develop the large number of polyps that people with FAP develop. However, most HNPCC cancers still develop from polyps. HNPCC is a much more common problem than FAP, accounting for 3% to 5% of all colorectal cancer. Like FAP, it is an autosomal dominant condition so that each child, regardless of gender, has a 50% chance of inheriting the gene mutation from the affected parent. The average age for colorectal cancer in HNPCC is 44 years. This is younger than the average of 64 years in sporadic (non-genetic) colorectal cancer, but older than in patients with FAP. Individuals with an HNPCC gene mutation have an estimated 70% lifetime risk of developing colorectal cancer, as opposed to the 100% chance that FAP patients have.

HNPCC is also associated with the development of other cancers including cancer of the uterus, ovary, small bowel, ureter, liver, bile ducts, and brain (Table 8). The most common associated cancer is cancer of the lining of the uterus (endometrium).

TABLE 8. RISKS OF TYPES OF CANCER IN HNPCC VERSUS GENERAL POPULATION.

TYPE OF CANCER	RISK IN HNPCC CARRIER	RISK IN GENERAL POPULATION
Colorectal cancer (men and women)	80%	6%
Endometrial (uterus) cancer	30–60%	2%
Ovarian cancer	10–12%	1–2%
Other cancers—stomach, small bowel, kidney, pancreas, urinary tract	slight increase	less than 2%

The family tree illustrated by Figure 33 depicts the kind of family history that would suggest HNPCC. What you notice in this family is a pattern of cancer, starting with the grandmother who died (slash mark) of colorectal cancer in her 50s. Three of her sons also had colorectal cancer (two of them died of it), and one daughter died of cancer of the ovary. The other three siblings in that generation have not had cancer. We also see that in one son's family, two sons and a daughter have had colorectal cancer and another daughter had endometrial cancer (cancer of the uterus lining). One does not need to be an expert in genetics to notice that this family has a very strong and unusual history of cancer. The specific features of this family history that suggest HNPCC include colorectal cancer in several closely related people on one side of the family (seven relatives over three generations), colorectal cancers diagnosed at younger ages than usual (three were diagnosed in their 40s), and other cancers that are known to be more common with the syndrome (e.g., endometrial and ovarian cancer).

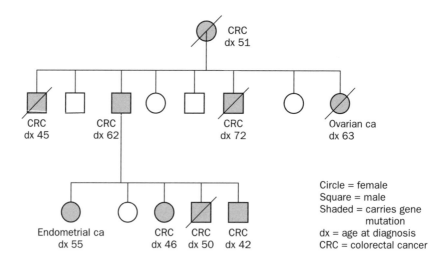

Figure 33. *An HNPCC family history.*

The specific criteria for defining an HNPCC family are known as the *Amsterdam Criteria II*. For an individual to be diagnosed as having HNPCC, all of the following must apply:

- The individual's family must include at least three relatives with colorectal cancer or an HNPCC-associated cancer.
- One individual is a *first-degree* (immediate) *relative* of the other two.
- At least two successive generations are affected.
- At least one member was diagnosed with cancer before the age of 50.
- FAP has been excluded in the colorectal cancer cases.
- The cancers have been verified by a formal laboratory examination.

HNPCC is caused by a mutation of one of several DNA damage repair (mismatch repair) genes. The function of these genes is to make sure that DNA (the genetic material) does not get corrupted or damaged when cells divide. They act like the "spell check" in a computer program. The genes MSH2 at chromosome band 2p16 and MLH1 at chromosome band 3p21 are the two most important genes relating to HNPCC. Genetic testing is available to search for mutations in MSH2 and MLH1, but at least two other genes can also cause HNPCC, so this testing may not provide answers in all cases.

In patients whose families fit the Amsterdam Criteria II, genetic testing will show positive results for an MSH2 or MLH1 gene mutation in up to 25% of cases. If a mutation is identified in an affected person, testing for that same mutation could be offered to family members at risk.

Guidelines for screening in HNPCC

Screening for HNPCC must take into account how these colorectal cancers differ from non-hereditary colorectal cancers. HNPCC cancers appear at younger ages than sporadic colorectal cancers (15% of HNPCC patients develop colorectal cancer in their 40s), they more often arise from flat adenomas that may not be well seen on a barium enema, they more often occur in the right colon (60% to 70% of HNPCC cancers occur in the right colon), they may grow more rapidly, and affected people may develop other cancers (20% of HNPCC mutation carriers develop non-colorectal cancers by the age of 70, especially cancer of the uterus). These differences suggest that screening should begin early and should be carried out by colonoscopy. Because of the risk of endometrial cancer, the lining of the uterus should also be examined on a regular basis beginning at the age of 25.

Screening will vary depending on whether an HNPCC gene mutation is known to be present or absent (based upon genetic testing), or if the person has not undergone genetic testing.

If genetic testing shows the presence of the HNPCC gene, screening should include:

- ► Yearly colonoscopy beginning at age 25.
- ► Possibly, yearly examination of the uterus lining beginning at age 25. There has been some recent controversy as to whether such examination is of benefit. Patients should check with their physician.

If genetic testing shows the absence of the HNPCC gene:

- ► Screening should follow recommendations for the general population.

If the person has not had genetic testing, screening should include:

- ► Colonoscopy every one to two years from age 25 to 40, then yearly.
- ► Periodic uterine screening should be considered.

GENETIC TESTING AND GENETIC COUNSELING

The first step in identifying hereditary colorectal cancer is a careful assessment of the family history. This is usually done by a genetic counselor who works in a medical genetics or hereditary cancer clinic. When the family history suggests HNPCC or FAP, genetic testing may be able to identify a mutation in a specific gene associated with the cancer syndrome. This testing usually starts on a blood or tumor sample from a person in the family who has had cancer. This person is called the *index case*. If a specific gene mutation is found, then testing for that specific mutation is made available to other family members who wish to learn whether they have inherited that gene mutation and the associated cancer risks. If an otherwise well person in the family is found to have inherited the gene mutation, they will be advised to have careful cancer screening, as previously described. A family member who has been tested and found not to have inherited the gene mutation is at no greater risk for cancer than the general population, so only standard screening is recommended.

It is possible that no mutation will be found when genetic testing is done on the index case. Not all known gene mutations can be tested for, and there are likely some mutations that have not yet been discovered.

To test or not to test

Although it may seem like a simple decision, the benefits, risks, and limitations of genetic testing can be complex. One important thing to remember is that genes are shared with parents, brothers, sisters, children, and other relatives. This means that the results of genetic testing provide information about the family, not just oneself. Not everyone who might be eligible will choose to have genetic testing. Some people simply do not want to know. Others are worried about how a positive result could affect them socially or how it could potentially cause problems when applying for future health or life insurance. For these reasons, anyone who is considering genetic testing is strongly encouraged to meet with a genetic counselor before any blood samples go to a lab.

A genetic counseling appointment includes:

▸ Review and interpretation of the family history of cancer.

▸ Review of basic genetics, cancer genes, and related cancer risks.

▸ Recommendations for cancer screening based on the family history.

▸ Discussion about genetic testing—Is it possible? If so, how is it done? What are the risks, benefits, and limitations?

▸ Discussion about sharing this information with family members.

With the support of appropriate genetic counseling, FAP genetic testing can be done for children with a suggestive personal or family history because of the implications for their cancer screening. HNPCC testing, however, is only offered to adults because cancer screening for HNPCC does not need to begin in childhood. If you have a family history that looks like the examples in this chapter, you should talk to your doctor about a referral for genetic risk assessment. Such services are available in most provinces and states. You may also want to talk with other relatives to find out if anyone else has already looked into this.

Should genetic testing be done on everyone routinely?

People whose family histories do not suggest a hereditary pattern of cancer are not generally recommended to have genetic testing at this time. The rarity of inherited mutations in the APC and HNPCC-associated genes in such individuals combined with the current cost of testing and the fact that not all mutations can be identified, makes general population testing potentially misleading and not cost effective.

FAMILIAL COLORECTAL CANCER (FCC)

Ten to fifteen percent of patients with colorectal cancer or adenomas have other affected family members. However, their family histories do not fit the criteria for either FAP or HNPCC, and may not appear to follow a recognizable pattern of inheritance, such as autosomal dominant inheritance. Such families are categorized as having *familial colorectal cancer* (FCC). This may be due to genetic factors that have not yet been discovered, shared environmental risk, or even chance.

An estimated 7% to 10% of people have a first-degree relative with colorectal cancer, and twice that many have either a first-degree or second-degree relative with colorectal cancer. When you have a family history of colorectal cancer, the risk of getting it yourself is increased earlier in life rather than later. As a person with a family history ages beyond 50, his or her cancer risk begins to decline toward that of the normal population. Individuals with a personal history of an adenomatous polyp have a 15% to 20% risk of developing a subsequent polyp. A history of adenomatous polyps in a sibling or parent is associated with an increased risk of polyps and colorectal cancer. If you have a history of polyps or colorectal cancer in your family, be sure to bring it to the attention of your family doctor.

RARE POLYP/COLORECTAL CANCER SYNDROMES

MUIR-TORRE SYNDROME

A variant of HNPCC that includes skin lesions and colorectal cancer.

TURCOT SYNDROME

Turcot syndrome includes colorectal polyps, colon cancer, and brain tumors. This may be a variant of FAP or HNPCC.

PEUTZ-JEHGERS SYNDROME

This syndrome is characterized by black freckles on the lips, gums and anus, as well as multiple intestinal polyps, both adenomas and hamartomas (see Chapter 6 for information on the various kinds of polyps).

JUVENILE POLYPOSIS SYNDROME

This syndrome is characterized by hamartomas throughout the gastrointestinal tract in childhood, as well as diarrhea, bleeding, and loss of proteins from the bowel.

WHAT IS A STOMA?

A *stoma* is an opening on the abdominal wall where the severed end of the intestine is sewn to the skin. Its purpose is to divert the flow of feces. The intestinal contents pass out through the stoma and into an *appliance* (collecting bag or pouch). *Ostomy* is a term interchangeable with stoma.

A stoma can be created anywhere on the abdomen and any part of the bowel may be used for this. The site of the stoma and the part of bowel used for the stoma are determined by the individual characteristics of each patient's abdomen and disease.

LOOP VERSUS END

There are two basic stoma configurations: loop stoma and end stoma. A *loop stoma* is created by making a side-hole in the intestine that is sewn to the edges of an abdominal wall opening. The bowel is not divided. An *end stoma*, on the other hand, requires complete division of the bowel (Figure 34). The upper end is brought through the abdominal wall and is sewn to the opening to create an end stoma. The lower end is often sewn over and left within the abdominal cavity. If the lower end of the bowel is brought out through a separate opening, that stoma is called a *mucus fistula*.

A loop stoma is used when there is a temporary need for a diversion of feces. It allows the bowel beyond the stoma to be rested (the stool will pass out into the appliance rather than continuing to go further down the intestinal tract) and has the advantage of being very easy to close during a subsequent operation. The drawback of a loop stoma, however, is that it is prone to prolapse (create a protrusion) and is more difficult to care for because it is not round and appliances often do not fit it as well as they do an end stoma.

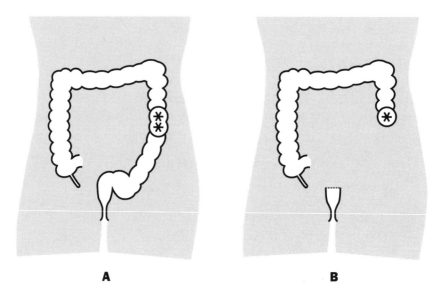

A   **B**

Figure 34. *Loop (A) and end (B) stomas.*

COLOSTOMY VERSUS ILEOSTOMY

If the large intestine (colon) is used to make a stoma, it is called a *colostomy* (Figure 35). A colostomy may be either a loop colostomy or an end colostomy. Since the contents are large intestinal contents, the feces that come from a colostomy resemble typical bowel movement material. Although there is no control over when a stoma drains, a colostomy tends to "act" once or twice a day, usually at about the same time each day. There is no sphincter muscle to control when the colostomy will function.

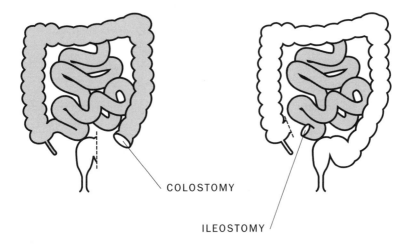

COLOSTOMY

ILEOSTOMY

Figure 35. *Colostomy and ileostomy.*

Some individuals with a colostomy may choose to irrigate the colostomy. This is like giving yourself an enema and should be taught by an enterostomal therapist after the physician has approved of the patient managing the colostomy in this manner. The advantage of irrigating a colostomy is that it gives the patient more control over when the colostomy will empty.

If the small intestine is used to make a stoma, it is called an *ileostomy*. An ileostomy (Figure 35) may be either a loop ileostomy or an end ileostomy. The material that comes from an ileostomy is small intestinal contents and is green rather than brown. Initially it may be quite watery, but it will thicken to the consistency of toothpaste. An ileostomy drains more frequently and irregularly than a colostomy.

WHEN ARE STOMAS REQUIRED?

A stoma is required under the following circumstances:

AS PART OF AN ABDOMINOPERINEAL OPERATION FOR LOWER THIRD RECTAL CANCER (SEE CHAPTER 21)

When a cancer in the lower third of the rectum is removed by an abdomino-perineal resection, the entire anus is taken with the specimen and the anal area sewn closed. The end of the colon is then brought out through an opening that is made in the abdominal wall. The end of the bowel is sewn to the edges of the opening and stool then passes through the bowel and out the stoma. Since this stoma is made from the colon it is called a colostomy. As there is no longer any anus after an abdominoperineal resection, the colostomy is permanent.

TO PROTECT AN ANASTOMOSIS

When a segment of cancerous bowel is removed, the remaining ends are stapled back together. The joint is called an anastomosis. Normally, an anastomosis will heal quickly and stool and gas will pass through it in the usual way. Occasionally, an anastomosis will leak within a week or two of surgery. This is a potentially life-threatening complication. Sometimes a surgeon will decide to take steps to prevent this from happening by making an upstream stoma to protect the anastomosis. This is usually a loop stoma. The value of this diverting stoma is that it gives the anastomosis extra time to heal by preventing any stool or gas from getting down to it. Once the patient is recovering well from the operation, say at three months, the stoma can be closed at a second operation.

Certain conditions will give a surgeon concern that the risk for anastomotic leak is higher than normal and will increase the chance that the patient will awake from surgery with a stoma. These conditions include:

- A malnourished, ill, or frail patient.

- A colon that has been obstructed (blocked) by a cancer.
- The presence of infection in the abdomen.
- A difficult or very low rectal anastomosis.

SELECTION OF STOMA SITE

It is important that the location of the stoma site on the abdominal wall be carefully chosen. An improperly placed stoma can interfere significantly with the patient's ability to get back to a full and active life. Ideally, an enterostomal therapist (an experienced nurse trained in the management of stomas) should choose the site before surgery. The enterostomal therapist assesses the patient's lifestyle, occupation, hobbies, sports, and favored dress style and selects the stoma site so as to cause minimal interference with these activities. Wrinkles or scars on the abdominal wall, the position of folds that appear during bending and sitting, poor eyesight, diminished manual dexterity, and special needs such as wheelchair or crutches are also taken into account when determining the best possible stoma site.

In most cases, the stoma is placed below the waist, on the left or right as dictated by the operation. It is usually located within eight cm (three inches) of the centerline of the abdomen so that it passes through one of the two rectus muscles (Figure 36). These muscles provide the stoma with strong muscular support. It is important for the stoma to lie on a flat area of the abdomen. If it is too close to irregularities created by bony prominences from ribs, hip bones, or the pubic bone, or near the belly-button, it will be difficult to maintain a good seal between the appliance and the skin.

Once the final location is selected, an indelible mark is placed on the chosen site so that it can be easily identified during surgery.

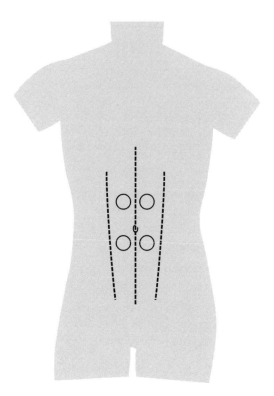

Figure 36. *Potential stoma sites.*

SELECTION AND CARE OF OSTOMY EQUIPMENT

There have been many improvements to the ostomy appliances of the 1950s when thick, cumbersome, odorous rubber pouches cemented to the skin with surgical adhesive or simple wads of dressings were the only options available. Manufacturers have listened to enterostomal therapists, doctors, and patients who demanded something better. Intensive research has led to the development of hypoallergenic products, adhesives that are gentle to the skin, and appliances that offer improved security and comfort.

Two types of stoma appliance systems are currently available: two-piece systems and one-piece systems (Figure 37).

TWO-PIECE SYSTEM

The first part of the two-piece system is the flange, which consists of a plastic ring mounted on an adhesive skin barrier. The second part of the system is the collecting pouch that snaps onto the plastic ring of the flange. Pouches come in a variety of sizes and shapes. They have a grooved ring on the back surface that corresponds to the ring on the flange. The two rings clamp together, much like the lid on a Tupperware container.

The two-piece system can be customized by the patient. Using a pattern guide found to be the best personal fit, the wearer uses a pair of scissors to cut out a hole in the flange to fit the stoma. Alternatively, pre-cut flanges of various sizes are available for those who do not wish to cut their own. There are also hole cutters available, which are something like a cookie cutter to assist in cutting the proper size opening when shrinkage has been completed (there will be some shrinkage of the stoma in the first six weeks after surgery).

Two-piece systems come with either an open end (which is closed with a tail clip, designed for those who must empty the pouch frequently), or a closed pouch (which is meant for one-time use, designed for those who have only one or two colostomy movements per day).

An important advantage of the two-piece system is that the pouch can be removed from the flange without disturbing the skin; the flange remains in place. For this reason, many people prefer the two-piece system even though it is a little more complicated to apply. It is of particular advantage to those who have to empty more frequently, or who wish to alternate from a larger pouch during the night to a smaller one during the day or when swimming, etc. Mini-pouches are available for such instances. It should be noted that a mini-pouch has less capacity and doesn't reach down as far as the standard pouch when one is seated on the toilet to empty it. The flange may be left in place for up to seven days, depending on the preference and activities of the user.

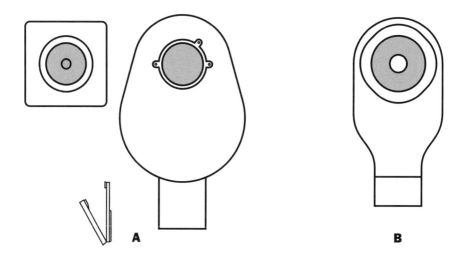

Figure 37. *A. Two-piece system—separate flange (square) stays on the skin when pouch is removed. B. One-piece system—flange is part of pouch.*

ONE-PIECE SYSTEM

The one-piece system combines the skin barrier, flange, and collecting pouch into a single unit. The pouches can be purchased with a pre-cut opening or in a custom cut version that allows the user to customize the opening.

One-piece pouches also come with either an open end or a closed pouch.

One-piece systems are easy to put on and lie very flat, so they are well hidden under clothing. When a change is required, the entire appliance is removed and disposed of and a new one applied on the skin.

Many one-piece systems have gas vents incorporated into the pouch. The vent includes an activated charcoal filter that deodorizes the gas as it passes through. The advantage of the vent is that it permits longer wearing of the one-piece unit, which would otherwise have to be entirely removed when it has filled with gas. These work best for colostomies. When using a pouch with a gas vent, to make it effective, you must wear clothing that is fairly snug-fitting in order to force the gas out of the pouch. With loose clothing, it will blow up like a balloon. The more watery drainage of an ileostomy often clogs the valve. A vent is not as critical in the two-piece system because the seal between the flange and the pouch can be opened at any time to "burp" the pouch.

CARE AND MANAGEMENT OF A STOMA

Other than the closed-end one-piece system, appliances can be worn for four to seven days. Seven days is ideal for most people. The first step in putting on a new one is removing the old one. When doing so, take care not to damage the skin when peeling off the tape and adhesive layer. Appliances are made of lightweight plastic and therefore should not be disposed of down a toilet. Instead, wrap them in newspaper and dispose of them in the garbage. Most people keep a small zip-lock bag in their ostomy kit bag for disposal of soiled pouches in public facilities. The pouch can be wrapped in toilet tissue, put into the zip-lock bag, and then into the washroom garbage receptacle. Pouches should be rinsed out before disposal. Plastic pouches containing stool should not be sent to landfill sites. It is easier to use a drainable pouch so it doesn't have to be disposed of in a public washroom or someone else's home.

Once you have removed the appliance, wash the skin around the stoma with warm water—some people like to take a bath or a shower at this stage, but remember you do not always know when the stoma is going to function. Use just water, as chemical ingredients found in some soaps can be irritating to the stoma and drying to the skin. Remove residual adhesive material, carefully inspect the skin, and take corrective action if you see redness or irritation. If you have hair under the appliance, you need to be very careful about shaving. You should not use a straight-edge razor, which can cause small nicks and spread bacteria. Instead, use an electric razor or cut the hair with scissors. You may also consider a chemical depilatory provided it does not cause irritation or allergy to the skin. Electrolysis is also another option, provided it is done by a skilled professional. Because this may cause local injury to the skin, topical antimicrobial coverage with an alcohol lotion would be a good idea after electrolysis and prior to applying the appliance. If there is any soapy residue, wash it off, and then pat it dry.

In the early weeks, you should measure the stoma before applying a pouch because there is some shrinkage and the appliance opening must continue to fit appropriately. Most shrinkage will be completed within six weeks of the surgery. The appliance should fit with just a hairline space around the stoma but the edges must not be allowed to touch the fragile mucus membrane of the stoma.

If you need it, you can use a skin sealant for skin protection. Barrier film comes in a liquid form packaged in small tissue packs. The wet tissue is simply wiped onto the skin surrounding the stoma and the fluid is permitted to dry to a plastic-like layer. If you have an oily texture to your skin, these can sometimes help the adhesion of the appliance, but are not necessary for most people.

The principle on which the skin barrier works is that body heat softens it and makes it tacky so that it can adhere to the skin. When using a sealant, this process takes longer. If you require skin sealant to protect against the adhesive part of the flange or to make it easier to remove, it should just be put under the adhesive area. Sealants are also available in spray or roll-on.

Fill any skin creases with ostomy paste, or you can apply the paste directly to the edges of the stoma opening of the flange to provide an extra seal. Line up the opening of the flange with the stoma and press the flange into place.

If you need a more durable seal around the base of the stoma, there are barrier strips that you can use by wrapping them around the stoma, or there are barrier rings that you can use that don't deteriorate as quickly as the paste or the skin barrier on the flange. The strip or ring replaces the paste.

Many flanges already have tape on them, so it should not be necessary to use additional tape, but if you feel you need extra protection, hypoallergenic tape is placed around the edges of the flange like a picture frame. Waterproof tape should not be used because it often leads to skin irritation. However, there is now a silicone tape with no adhesive on it, which is waterproof and can be used for extra reassurance. Belts are also available for extra security, but most people don't use them.

LIFE WITH A STOMA

PERSONAL RELATIONSHIPS

While most patients learn the basic skills of changing their appliance before leaving the hospital, the first few days at home can be difficult. Many people experience anxiety as they try to adjust to the change in their bodies, to the loss of support of hospital staff, and to the reintegration into their circle of family and friends. The time required for adjustment varies. It is a good idea for a partner, friend, or family member to be included in the ostomy-management teaching at the hospital so that he or she can become familiar with stoma drainage, skin care, and equipment. This person can provide invaluable support at home during the early phase of convalescence. Other important early support services include visits from a home care nurse, homemaker services, and perhaps a contact member of the local chapter of the United Ostomy Association.

It usually takes at least three months following abdominal surgery for normal strength to return. With it comes confidence in living with and caring for the stoma, and the feeling of self-respect and well-being. Most non-exertional hobbies and work can be resumed as soon as you feel up to it. There is no pursuit that a person with a stoma cannot undertake if the will is there, although during the first three months it is best to avoid activities that require heavy lifting or straining, in order to allow the wounds time to heal.

SEXUAL ACTIVITIES

Loss of energy, weakness in the early postoperative period, on-going cancer treatments, or pain in the healing area can all initially interfere with a return to sexual activity. Sometimes impotence may occur as a result of the surgery (see Chapter 23). Women may find that intercourse can be painful after surgery. However, as far as the stoma is concerned, most people are able to resume sexual activity when health and energy return.

Probably the most important factors in good sexual relationships are an ability to communicate and a good sense of humor. For the person with a stoma, however, some preparation is helpful if sexual activity is contemplated, and good hygiene is essential. A person wearing a two-piece system might wish to change to a smaller pouch, or to empty and clean the pouch, perhaps taping it for extra security before sexual activity.

WORK, TRAVEL, AND SPORTS

Returning to a full, satisfying life needs a little planning. It is useful to carry a small cosmetic or shaving bag filled with supplies for an emergency appliance change. This can be kept inconspicuously in a briefcase, purse, pocket, or glove compartment of the car.

Returning to work is usually a boost to the morale, but care should be taken not to overdo things at the beginning.

A stoma should not interfere with travel. Although ostomy equipment is available world wide, types or designs may differ between continents. It is a good idea to check with the enterostomal therapist or the United Ostomy Association about resources available at your destination. In addition, pack twice as much equipment as you think you will need, and be sure to carry it in your hand luggage!

In areas where the water supply is not clean, be careful—diarrhea and stomas are an unhappy mix. Water-purifying tablets and a prescription for antidiarrheal medication can be handy travel companions. Also, keep in mind that warm climates and exertion reduce the wearing time of the appliance and greater care and more frequent changes will be needed.

Sports are fun as well as physically and psychologically healthy, and there is really no sport that is out of bounds. Obviously, special care is needed for body-contact sports like wrestling, which can traumatize the stoma or dislodge the appliance. Sport shields are available for contact sports.

If a peristomal hernia should develop, there are hernia support belts that can be fitted to help give support. These should be fitted by a qualified professional.

DIET

Most people with colostomies resume a normal diet without difficulty as the major part of their digestive tract is still intact. Often, diet counseling will be provided in the hospital prior to your discharge. Some patients find that certain foods alter their stoma function and adapt by making appropriate changes. Some experimentation is required to determine whether certain items should be avoided. You can drink alcoholic beverages in moderation, although some people find they cause gas and looser bowel movements. Grape juice and prune juice can have similar effects. Sometimes, the addition of these substances to the diet during periods of constipation can be helpful. By such means, you will learn to best regulate your stoma.

For the first four to six weeks after surgery, it is generally recommended that a patient with an ileostomy be restricted to a diet low in roughage. Eat well cooked, soft foods, and avoid fresh vegetables and popcorn. Then start to gradually introduce new foods in small quantities to make certain that there is no problem with digestion through the small bowel.

People who have ileostomies have lost the benefit of the water-absorbing function of the large intestine and therefore produce more watery stool. They must learn to replace lost fluid and, to some extent, lost sodium and potassium. Drainage can be thickened by foods such as apple sauce, bananas, peanut butter, or rice. A bulk-forming agent such as Metamucil can also be very useful for thickening the stool. Most foods have sodium in them, but you may want to add a little extra unless there is a specific medical reason to avoid it. Foods high in potassium such as bananas, tomatoes, and oranges should be included in the diet. Gastrolyte or other special electrolyte-balanced drinks help replace fluid, potassium, and sodium. These drinks are found in pharmacies and are preferable to Gatorade, which contains a high volume of sugar that can cause diarrhea.

GAS AND ODOR

If you have a colostomy or ileostomy, you will probably have problems with gas and odor at one time or another. Some food culprits are cabbage, broccoli, beans, beer, and some highly spiced foods, but judicious consumption can control the problem. Yogurt, buttermilk, and parsley can actually help to diminish odor. Smoking, chewing gum, drinking soda drinks, using a straw, talking while eating, skipping meals, and sleeping with your mouth open can lead to air ingestion and extra gas.

There are many commercial products available to counteract odor. Some can be taken orally, others can be put directly into the pouch. The most commonly used deodorants are unscented liquids that are put into the pouch after emptying as they will coat the inside of the pouch and come in contact with the discharge immediately. If you are thinking of using an oral deodorant, talk to your physician to make certain that it doesn't interfere with any other medication. Since today's appliances are odor-proof, there is no reason why odor should be a problem provided the stoma and appliances are well-managed.

Caution: Some complementary agents or therapies may be useful for cancer patients; however, some may be harmful in certain situations. Intelligent Patient Guide Ltd. cautions you to consult with your oncologist before attempting to use any agents or therapies mentioned on these pages. Inclusion of an agent, therapy, or resource in this chapter does not imply endorsement by Intelligent Patient Guide Ltd.

WHAT DO THE TERMS ALTERNATIVE AND COMPLEMENTARY MEAN?

Alternative therapy means treatment that is different from standard medical practice. *Complementary therapy* refers to treatment that is designed to supplement standard medical practice.

ALTERNATIVE THERAPY

Mainstream treatment for cancer is called conventional therapy. It means that the value of the treatment has been demonstrated by rigorous scientific testing and is given by physicians who are licensed by regulated colleges of medicine. If these treatments worked 100% of the time, there would be no need for alternative therapies. Unfortunately, conventional therapy for cancer does not always work, so the opportunity for alternative treatments arises. Alternative therapies may involve anything from dietary supplements to elaborate and expensive therapies at private clinics in foreign countries.

The term *alternative* may not be appropriate since it implies an element of equivalency, which is rarely justified. A more appropriate label might be *unproven therapies* or *questionable therapies*, but for the purposes of this chapter, they will be called alternative therapy.

COMPLEMENTARY THERAPY

Therapies that add to or support conventional treatment are said to be complementary. They may include psychological counseling, biofeedback, meditation, massage, and so on. Complementary treatments do not involve the use of drugs or invasive measures. They are not designed to cure cancer but to enhance the patient's general well-being and sense of control during the difficult stages of treatment and follow-up.

THE APPEAL OF ALTERNATE THERAPIES

The appeal that alternate therapies have for patients coping with cancer is understandable; 10% of cancer patients try them. This is a serious disease, and it seems sensible to try anything that appears to offer hope for cure. This is particularly the case if the disease does not appear to be responding to conventional therapy. In addition, many people today wish to take a more hands-on approach to their care, and alternative therapies give them an opportunity to do that, restoring some sense of control.

Poor outcome from conventional treatment can result in frustration and anger and even lead some to believe that the medical establishment and pharmaceutical companies are somehow narrowing treatment choices in an effort to monopolize treatment markets for the sake of professional status or financial gain. But no ethical doctor would deny patients access to any legal therapy that was shown to provide at least some benefit, and so such claims ring hollow to those who understand just how many thousands of scientists throughout the world are working away on the problem of beating cancer with little regard to personal benefit.

There is no doubt, however, that doctors' attitudes toward alternative treatment have played a role in enhancing the appeal of therapy. While the conventional physician rambles on about double-blind randomized studies and continues to prescribe unpleasant treatments, many patients start to wonder, what about me and my needs? Until recently, conventional medicine has been very weak in taking into account the importance of personal support, good nutrition, exercise, and mental attitudes during cancer care. Promoters of alternative therapies recognize this and fill this void by bringing holistic elements to their treatments, appealing to the whole person, in body and mind.

THE PROBLEM WITH ALTERNATIVE AND
COMPLEMENTARY THERAPIES

The primary concerns of physicians are that these treatments could worsen the colorectal cancer problem or interfere with or usurp conventional therapy that has been proven to do some good. No one disagrees that sound nutrition, exercise, relaxation, and psychological and spiritual support are important to the cancer patient. They can significantly improve quality of life and reduce the suffering that one experiences with cancer. But none of the alternative or complementary therapies, in the absence of conventional therapy, will stop colorectal cancer from progressing.

A METHOD FOR EVALUATING AN ALTERNATIVE THERAPY

Conventional treatment becomes conventional only after it has been subjected to years of research and rigorous evaluation. Before treatments are approved by the FDA in the United States or by Health Canada, an enormous amount of work has been done to prove the value of the treatment, and this work has been vetted by circumspect and impartial scientists. Even after approval, research is continued to further assess the treatment's therapeutic claims and to ensure that it performs within a range of safety that justifies its continued use. This rigorous testing and continued evaluation is not applied to alternative therapies.

Before you or a loved one undertakes an alternative treatment, consider the following questions as a means of evaluating the therapy:*

▸ Has the treatment been evaluated in clinical trials? Check with a librarian at a medical library in the nearest hospital.

▸ Do the promoters of the alternative therapy claim that the medical community is trying to keep their cure from the public? There is no greater indication of quackery than this.

▸ Does the treatment take place in a distant country? This puts practitioners in these clinics outside of the range of demanding North American regulators.

▸ Does it involve a claim that a nutritional or dietary therapy can cure cancer? At this time, there is no known dietary cure for cancer.

▸ Do the promoters say that it is harmless and produces no side effects? Even a sugar pill has side effects if one carefully analyzes its effects. Such side effects must be accurately measured and documented for Health Canada or FDA approval. Because treatments for cancer must

*Adapted from The National Cancer Institute

be powerful, the medicines that show promise of working have side effects. If a treatment is promoted as having no side effects, either there has been no formal testing done or the promoter is ignorant of accepted testing procedures or is misrepresenting or unaware of results. None of these possibilities is good.

▶ Is it a secret formula that only a small group of practitioners can use? In the real world of medicine, scientists publish their results so they can be evaluated and validated by the general scientific community. Whoever discovers the cure for cancer will win the Nobel Prize and will be remembered for all time; there is no Nobel Prize given for secrecy in medicine.

TYPES OF ALTERNATIVE AND COMPLEMENTARY THERAPIES

Alternative and complementary therapies can be grouped into the following categories:

Folk
- herbal medicine
- homeopathic medicine

Nutritional
- diet supplements
- macrobiotics
- megavitamins
- fasting therapy
- juice therapy
- Gerson/coffee enemas

Mind/body control
- biofeedback
- guided imagery
- hypnotherapy
- music/sound therapy
- relaxation therapy

Pharmacological and biological
- cartilage
- melatonin
- selenium
- ozone
- pancreatic enzymes
- antioxidants
- chelation therapy

Structural manipulations/ energetic therapies
- acupuncture
- accupressure
- chiropractic medicine
- electromagnetic

Qi gong and Tai chi reflexology
- Rolfing
- therapeutic touch

The range of alternative therapies is vast and is continually increasing. Brief descriptions of some of these therapies are included below. The source for this information is The University of Texas M.D. Anderson Cancer Center. More information can be obtained from their web site at www.mdanderson.org.

HOMEOPATHIC THERAPY

The practice of homeopathy is based on its proposed "law of similars," which suggests that "like cures like." That is, a substance that causes specific symptoms in a healthy person could cure those same symptoms in a sick person. Homeopathic medicines are intended to enable the body to initiate the healing process, rather than eliminate the symptom. No direct anti-tumor mechanism of action has been proposed. Furthermore, the traditional method for developing homeopathic medicines involves producing symptoms in healthy persons so this would be unthinkable in the context of causing tumors. A proposed secondary role to support the overall health of the patient with cancer has not been established at this time.

Homeopathic medicines are traditionally very small doses of natural substances that have been diluted in water or alcohol many times and are generally taken orally.

Side effects may vary with the individual, but these are rarely identified in articles aimed at patients with cancer. Although homeopathic medicines are highly diluted, some of them do include toxic substances such as Aristolochia. Negative results have been reported when homeopathic treatment was substituted for conventional cancer treatment.

MACROBIOTICS

The macrobiotic diet is part of ancient Asian philosophy that attempts to achieve balance between the opposing forces that exist in the universe (yin and yang). According to macrobiotic theory, certain foods are yin and others are yang, and certain cancers are yin while others are yang. The aim is to consume foods that balance against the type of cancer one has.

According to this way of thinking, foods such as sugar, citrus fruits, and spices are classified as yin while animal foods are classified as yang. Breast cancer is a yin cancer and so the opposite, or yang, foods should be consumed by such patients. Colon cancer, on the other hand, is classified according to macrobiotic theory as a yang cancer so followers are advised to consume more yin foods. A diet for colon cancer calls for milder seasoning, more light cooking, and more leafy green vegetables.

Claims that a macrobiotic diet can prevent or treat cancer have been made, but have never been scientifically proven. Furthermore, studies have found that adults following a macrobiotic diet had an average intake of only 60% to 70% of the recommended daily intake of calories. A macrobiotic diet typically does not provide enough of certain nutrients, such as protein, to provide balanced nutrition. Macrobiotic diet calls for 50% to 60% rice and whole-grain cereals, 20% to 25% vegetables, and 5% to 10% beans and sea vegetables. The diet is thought to be nutritionally unsound by many nutritional scientists. Many people who eat such a diet lose weight. This is a problem for people with cancer since weight loss may impair the ability to tolerate certain treatments and complications and is generally associated with poorer outcome from cancer.

GERSON PROGRAM

The Gerson program is one of the oldest Western nutritional approaches to cancer treatment. German physician, Max B. Gerson, developed it in the 1940s. The critical elements of this program are the balance of sodium and potassium, high doses of micronutrients by frequent consumption of fruit and vegetable juices, strict dietary fat reduction, temporary restriction of protein with a vegetarian diet, and frequent coffee enemas. Studies have reported higher survival rates for patients with melanoma, colorectal, and ovarian cancers who participated in the Gerson program compared to similar patients reported in the literature who did not participate in the program. In cases where no increase in survival has been reported, there is a tendency for improvement in general health and well-being. The program may last from a few months to 10 years.

Side effects include flu-like feelings, loss of appetite, weakness, dizziness, and perspiration with strong odor. Tumor masses may become painful, and patients may experience high fever, intestinal cramping, diarrhea, and vomiting. Although coffee enemas were used and endorsed as a detoxification regimen by the medical community until the early 1970s, there is controversy about the metabolic alterations they may produce. Coffee enemas may cause colitis (severe inflammation of the colon). The coffee enemas may also cause serious fluid and electrolyte problems in the body. Serious infections and deaths from electrolyte imbalance due to the use of coffee enemas have been reported.

CARTILAGE

Cartilage has been investigated since the 1950s for its properties of acceleration of wound healing and relief of arthritic pain. Potential properties of use in cancer treatment have included immune stimulation, antiangiogenesis (counteraction of new blood vessel formation), and protease inhibition (inhibition of certain invasive enzymes produced by tumors). Most of these investigations have been in animal studies, but a few human studies have been completed. Sophisticated studies are in process that may provide more definite conclusions concerning the value of cartilage in the treatment of cancer in humans.

Since cartilage may inhibit new blood vessel growth, caution is advised for anyone who is still growing and needs new blood vessel development, pregnant women, or individuals who are recovering from surgery or have cardiovascular problems. Because of the high content of calcium, it should not be taken by anyone with hypercalcemia or renal problems.

MELATONIN

Melatonin is a hormone produced by the pineal gland in the brain. It is activated by darkness and suppressed by light, so blood serum levels gradually increase after dark and peak after two a.m. Levels generally decline with age. Melatonin taken orally is derived from animals, but some herbs have trace amounts. It has been found to be effective for treatment of insomnia in humans and to modulate some components of the immune system. Protective effects against substances known to initiate or promote cancer have been demonstrated in animals and to some extent in humans. Studies in humans have included randomized clinical trials, but these trials were not blinded, so results may have been subject to bias. The one randomized trial that was blinded reported that melatonin did not have any demonstrated bone marrow protection effects for patients treated with chemotherapy.

Side effects include sleepiness in the day if melatonin is taken late at night. A few cases have been reported of negative effects for people with arthritis or taking warfarin (Coumadin).

ACUPUNCTURE

Acupuncture is a part of the health care systems of Asian countries such as China, Japan, Korea, and others. It can be traced back at least 2,500 years. The general theory is that patterns of energy/life flow exist in the body that are essential for health. Disruptions of these flow patterns are believed to be responsible for disease. Acupuncture seeks to correct imbalances of flow at identifiable points close to the skin by stimulation through a variety of techniques such as penetration of the skin by thin, solid, metallic needles, heat, or pressure.

A panel of independent experts convened by the National Institutes of Health (NIH) reviewed the clinical studies of acupuncture (many of which had been sponsored by the NIH). The panel first noted that the results of many studies were unclear because of poor study design, not enough patients, and other factors. The panel concluded that acupuncture has been shown to be effective for relief of adult postoperative nausea and vomiting, and chemotherapy-induced nausea and vomiting.

The most studied method is penetration of the skin by thin, solid, metallic needles, which are manipulated manually or stimulated electrically. Stimulation of these points by moxibustion (warming of certain herbs), pressure, heat, and lasers may also be used, but less information is available in the literature concerning these methods.

No side effects were noted in the NIH review. The occurrence of adverse events has been documented to be extremely low. However, these events have occurred on rare occasions (some of them life-threatening such as a collapsed lung from needles placed through the chest wall). The US Food and Drug Administration has removed acupuncture needles from the category of "experimental medical devices" and now regulates them as they do other devices such as surgical scalpels and hypodermic syringes. Credentials and licensing procedures for practitioners are regulated by individual provinces.

CHIROPRACTIC THERAPY

Manipulative and body-based therapies include osteopathic and chiropractic therapy. Although there may not be direct treatment effects upon the cancer, relief of various associated symptoms has been reported. Caution should be observed, particularly following surgery, radiation or chemotherapy, when joints and tissues may be inflamed or weakened and are easily damaged.

QI GONG AND TAI CHI

Qi gong (also spelled chee gung or chee koong) and Tai chi ch'uan (also spelled ty chee or taiji quan) are ancient practices of breathing, stretching, and slow-moving meditative postures that flow from one form to another. Both have been known by many different names throughout Chinese history. Qi gong is generally considered the more ancient system and many of its teachings are incorporated within Tai chi. The postures of both practices appear simple, but are quite precise. Many of the movements have been modeled after the movements of animals.

Controlled but non-randomized studies in China have reported potential benefits in survival, reduction of treatment side effects, and improvement in general health for patients with cancer and other health problems.

Sessions can last from 15 minutes to a few hours, and daily practice is recommended. Morning sessions are carried out in loose, comfortable clothing with bare feet, socks, or soft shoes. Styles of Qi gong and Tai chi differ from one school or instructor to another.

Although you can learn much about Qi gong and Tai chi from books and videos, some aspects of both can be harmful if practised incorrectly. That's why it's a good idea to seek at least occasional help from a Qi gong or Tai chi master who can guide you safely through the routines. If you have difficulty balancing, you should be cautious with these techniques. Begin under the supervision of a physical therapist or other knowledgeable health professional, or by using a chair or wall until your balance improves. In general, these are mild exercises that are safe for most people.

GARLIC

Garlic (*Allium sativum*) has been used for health purposes since biblical times, and is mentioned in the writings of ancient Hebrews, Babylonians, Romans, and Egyptians. The builders of the pyramids reportedly ate garlic for strength and endurance. It is a member of the lily family and is closely related to onions and chives.

Side effects include heartburn and gas. Because garlic is known to have some anti-clotting effects, if you are taking anticoagulant drugs, including ASA, you should check with your health care provider prior to beginning a regular garlic regimen. Garlic may also reduce blood sugar, so glucose control could be affected. There are no known problems with pregnant women taking garlic, but breast-feeding mothers should be aware that garlic may cause an altered flavor in breast milk.

GREEN TEA

Green tea, like black tea, is made from the leaves of the plant *Camellia sinesis* but differs from black tea in its preparation. The leaves used for green tea are steamed or pan-dried without fermentation, so the active substances within the leaves can retain their qualities. The tea is consumed by billions of people, not only as a satisfying beverage, but also to promote health. There is some evidence that green tea lowers total cholesterol levels and improves the cholesterol profile, reduces platelet stickiness, lowers blood pressure, and enhances the immune system. Studies in animals have reported that green tea polyphenols reduce the spread of cancer cells.

The most common side effects include insomnia or nervousness and irregularities in heart rate (from the caffeine). Women who are pregnant or breast-feeding should not consume green tea in large amounts. If you have an anxiety disorder or an irregular heartbeat, you should limit your intake to no more than two cups daily.

LAETRILE

Laetrile is the trade name for a naturally occurring substance, amygdalin, which is found in the pits of many fruits and in some plants. Cyanide, a breakdown product from amygdalin, has been proposed as the main anti-cancer component, although two other breakdown products, prunasin and benzaldehyde, have also been proposed as cancer cell inhibitors. According to the National Cancer Institute (NCI), laetrile, by itself, has shown little anti-cancer activity in animal studies, although some combinations containing laetrile have shown activity. No anticancer activity has been demonstrated in any human trials, including one phase-II clinical trial by the NCI. Laetrile is not approved by the FDA for use in the United States.

Side effects of laetrile in the NCI trial were sometimes, but not always, associated with high blood levels of cyanide, produced by the breakdown of laetrile in the body. These side effects included nausea, vomiting, headache, dizziness, mental dullness, and dermatitis. Other side effects of cyanide poisoning can also include low blood pressure, droopy upper eyelid, difficulty walking, fever, coma, and death. Cyanide poisoning is a greater risk when laetrile is taken by mouth because intestinal bacteria and some commonly eaten plants (e.g., celery, peaches, bean sprouts, and carrots) contain enzymes that can activate the release of cyanide from the laetrile.

CAT'S CLAW

Cat's claw, or *uncaria tomentosa*, also known as *Krallendorn* in European literature, is a plant that grows in the rain forests of the Andes Mountains, particularly in Peru. The Spanish name for it is Uña de gato. The name comes from the claw-like features of the plant vines, which resemble a cat's claw. The inner bark is the part used for medicinal purposes. It is used for a variety of ailments, including inflammation, rheumatism, gastric ulcers, tumors, dysentery, arthritis, to stimulate the immune system, and to promote wound healing. Whether it is effective for these problems is not really known. Cat's claw is available as a tincture, as capsules, tablets, elixirs, and as a cream. As well, it may be used as a tea. It can also be found mixed with other herbal therapies such as aloe.

This product should not be taken if you have an autoimmune disease, multiple sclerosis, or tuberculosis. In Europe, health care providers avoid combining this herb with hormonal drugs, insulin, or vaccines. Do not take this product if you are pregnant or breast-feeding. Cat's claw may block platelets from forming clots, so you should be cautious if you are already taking a medication, including ASA, which thins the blood.

ALOE VERA

Aloe vera is a succulent (a member of the cactus family) that originally comes from Africa, although it is currently grown almost everywhere. It has long, green, fleshy leaves with small spikes along the edges. When snapped off the plant, the sweet smelling, somewhat gooey, gel-like substance inside each leaf and the latex (the sticky residue left behind after the liquid from the gel has evaporated) can be used for a variety of purposes.

Traditionally, as well as currently, aloe gel has been used to soothe dry or damaged skin, treat minor cuts and burns, and the latex, which contains a substance called *emodin*, has been used for constipation. The root is sometimes used for colic. In some parts of the world, such as India, aloe is used to treat intestinal infections. Aloe may be able to help stimulate the immune system, and may also have an anti-inflammatory effect. Studies are currently underway to explore these effects.

Aloe can be used in several ways. Fresh leaf gel or store bought gel or cream (as in a cosmetic that contains aloe) can be applied directly to the skin. Aloe can also be purchased in capsule or liquid form in order to be taken by mouth, or in powder form, which can be reconstituted when needed. Aloe has not been approved by the FDA for intravenous use; it is illegal to give injections of aloe vera in the United States.

Aloe is generally regarded as safe for use on the skin, but it can be carcinogenic if combined with alcohol and sun exposure. It is *not* generally regarded as safe when used for constipation and can actually worsen the problem, or cause dependency, or bring about an electrolyte imbalance.

An allergic reaction to aloe is considered rare but possible. Pregnant women or those with irritable bowel syndrome should not take aloe internally as it may cause uterine stimulation.

PSYCHOLOGICAL APPROACHES

Many different psychological mind-body approaches may be used as a complementary therapy to support patients with cancer. These approaches may include education, individual and group counseling, cognitive behavioral therapy, communication skills training, self-esteem building, relaxation methods, meditation, coping mechanisms for pain control, hypnosis, music, drama, and art. Psychological therapies require an investment in time and energy that may compete with family or other activities. Patients should be aware that psychotherapy sessions led by inexperienced or inappropriately trained individuals can have unintended negative emotional consequences. However, if led by skilled, responsible individuals, these approaches can provide valuable support and comfort when combined with conventional medical treatment.

CHAPTER 45
CLINICAL RESEARCH: HOW IS IT DONE
AND SHOULD YOU PARTICIPATE?

WHY ARE CLINICAL STUDIES IMPORTANT?

As most patients quickly learn, there are a lot of unanswered questions about cancer. What is the cause? Or is there more than one cause? Can we prevent it? What new treatment or approach might give better results than we're getting right now? Is there some way of curing cancer permanently?

Research studies (also called *trials*) try to answer these and other questions. This is an ongoing process, with questions perpetually being asked, and researchers constantly looking for better ways of treating patients. Sometimes we forget that the treatments we now consider as "standard" for cancer (drugs, surgery, radiation) were at one time experimental. It is because patients with cancer have volunteered to participate in research studies that the current treatments are available.

WHAT ARE THE STEPS IN TESTING A NEW TREATMENT?

All potential treatments go through the same type of rigorous evaluation process that is required in testing a new drug.

New drug treatments begin in the laboratory. If extensive tests in test tubes and mice show that a new drug has potential in treating cancer, then it is tested in humans in a preliminary study called a *Phase I study* to check side effects and to establish a dose level at which side effects are acceptable. The drug is then tested in a small group of patients to determine its effect in controlling the cancer, a so-called *Phase II study*. In this phase, the question is, "Does the drug work at a dose that is safe in humans?" Phase I and II studies usually involve patients with advanced or metastatic cancer. If the results are still promising, the question then arises whether the new drug is better than the standard treatment. To determine this, a *Phase III study* is done in which patients are randomly selected for either the new or old treatment. If it is not known which treatment is superior, it is ethical to compare the treatments in consenting, volunteer patients with cancer.

Scientific studies such as these must follow rigid statistical processes to confirm that the information gained is reliable and valid. Patients must give their consent before they are included in any study.

Media reports about advances in understanding cancer or new treatments are often based on very preliminary data. Sometimes, a promising Phase II study or even an animal study may be reported as a breakthrough. This may be confusing for the public as well as for physicians. Until a new treatment can be confirmed to be both effective and superior to standard therapy in large studies, it cannot be recommended as the new standard of care. However, with persistence and with the participation of patient volunteers, new therapies are being introduced every year.

WHAT SHOULD I DO IF I'M ASKED TO BE PART OF A STUDY?

Participation in any study is strictly voluntary. If you are asked to consider enrolling in a study, you should understand why the study is being done, what is already known about the treatment's side effects and benefits, and what the alternatives are. Many Phase II and III trials use treatments that have been available for some time, so there may be considerable information available. On the other hand, it is important to understand that the primary aim of a Phase I trial is to define the side effects, since usually very few other patients have received this treatment.

Before any study is done, hospital ethics committees evaluate the research plan to ensure that the rights of the patients are protected and that the study is ethical in its design and implementation. These ethics committees always include members of the public. Informed consent must be obtained from each patient before enrolment in the study. This means that the researcher must carefully discuss the study with each potential participant, explaining the reasons for it, the risks and benefits, and other options the patient has in terms of treatment. Patients should not sign consent to participate unless they have had all their questions answered thoroughly.

Patients must feel free to decide what is in their own best interest, and must be comfortable in choosing to be part of a study. They should understand that their standard of care will not change if they subsequently decide to withdraw from the study.

It is through the commitment of thousands of patients participating in clinical research that many advances have been made in the treatment of cancer. Being part of a study gives some patients a feeling of empowerment as they know they are contributing to future improvements in the understanding and treatment of cancer. This partnership of doctors, patients, and researchers is one of our greatest weapons in fighting disease.

APPENDIX
BOWEL PREPARATION INSTRUCTIONS

Colonoscopy is a procedure in which the entire lining of the large intestine (colon) is examined visually by means of a long flexible instrument. If polyps or other abnormalities are found in the bowel during the procedure, the surgeon can often remove them through the instrument. Colonoscopy with polypectomy is one of the most powerful tools we have available for cancer prevention in modern medicine. The examination takes 15 to 60 minutes. Intravenous sedation is given to make the procedure better tolerated. While you will not be put to sleep, you will be drowsy during the procedure and for a period of time afterwards, so it is important that you arrange to be taken home by a friend or partner and not drive for the remainder of the day.

PREPARING FOR A COLONOSCOPY

SEVERAL DAYS BEFORE THE EXAMINATION: Go to the drugstore and purchase two bottles (300 ml [10 oz] each) of Citro-Mag (you will not need a prescription). Put the Citro-Mag into the refrigerator and chill for several hours.

TWO DAYS BEFORE YOUR PROCEDURE: After supper, start a strictly clear fluid diet. This means water, clear tea, clear coffee, consommé, Jell-O (avoid red), pop, juices without pulp, etc. Do not drink milk. Do not drink only water.

THE MORNING BEFORE YOUR PROCEDURE: At 8 am take one bottle (300 ml [10 oz]) of Citro-Mag and divide it into four equal portions. Drink a portion of the Citro-Mag and follow it with a full large drinking glass of juice. Repeat until the entire bottle of Citro-Mag is consumed—it is best to consume the entire bottle of Citro-Mag within 90 minutes. This will cause you to begin having bowel movements. Continue on a clear fluid diet and supplement with generous amounts of additional juice or Gatorade to prevent dehydration. A can of Boost (available at the drugstore) is permissible if you are very hungry. Some patients find that a Gravol tablet one hour prior to the Citro-Mag helps with prevent nausea during the preparation.

THE NIGHT BEFORE YOUR PROCEDURE: At 6 pm take a second bottle of Citro-Mag in the same way (including the large glasses of juice).

THE MORNING OF YOUR PROCEDURE: Take all of your normal medications with a sip of water early in the morning of your procedure unless instructed otherwise. Do not take a diabetic pill. Do not take insulin unless instructed otherwise (diabetic patients requiring insulin should obtain specific instructions on how to manage their insulin from their specialist). Clear fluids are permitted up to four hours prior to the procedure (avoid black coffee). Remain fasting (nothing by mouth) after that.

ABDOMINOPERINEAL RESECTION an operation in which both the rectum and anus are removed.

ADENOMA a benign polyp that has the potential to become a colorectal cancer.

ADENOCARCINOMA the type of cancer that occurs in the colon and rectum.

ADJUVANT THERAPY chemotherapy or radiotherapy given after surgery to enhance cure.

ALKALINE PHOSPHATASE an enzyme produced by the liver may be elevated in the blood if there are liver metastases.

ALTERNATIVE THERAPY a scientifically unproven treatment used instead of or along with standard medical therapy.

ANASTOMOSIS the point where two remaining ends of the bowel are joined after the cancerous section is removed.

ANASTOMOTIC STRICTURE a narrowing of the anastomosis.

ANTERIOR RESECTION when a portion of the rectum is removed and the remaining ends are joined.

ANUS the last inch of the rectum, surrounded by the sphincter muscles.

APPLIANCE a plastic device placed over a stoma to catch stool.

ASCENDING COLON the part of the colon going up the right side of the abdomen.

ATELECTASIS collapse of small air spaces in the lung after surgery. This is a common cause of postoperative fever.

AUTOSOMAL DOMINANT INHERITANCE a genetic pattern in which both males and females have a 50% chance of getting an inherited disorder.

BARIUM ENEMA an X-ray of the colon.

BENIGN GROWTH (or *benign tumor*) small, harmless lumps of cells.

BIOPSY a sample of tissue.

BOWEL PREPARATION (BOWEL PREP) a process of cleansing the colon of feces in preparation for colonoscopy or surgery.

BRACHYTHERAPY radiotherapy given by placement of radioactive beads into or adjacent to a cancer (as opposed to the more traditional external beam radiation given by a machine outside of the body).

CANCER a mass of cells that aggressively grow, divide, and spread without regard for the needs and limitations of the body.

CANCER FAMILY SYNDROME see *HNPCC*.

CARCINOEMBRYONIC ANTIGEN (CEA) a substance produced by many colorectal cancers. CEA level can be measured in the blood.

CARCINOMA see *adenocarcinoma*.

CARCINOMA-IN-SITU a very superficial, early cancer that has not yet penetrated into deeper tissues.

CARCINOMATOSIS PERITONEII widespread cancer cells growing on the surfaces of tissues within the abdomen.

CECUM the first part of the colon, in the right lower part of the abdomen.

CHEMOTHERAPY treatment of cancer with drugs.

COLON (also called the *large intestine*) the last major part of the digestive tract where waste material is formed into feces and held for elimination.

COLONOSCOPE flexible, 160 cm instrument designed for viewing the entire colon and rectum.

COLONOSCOPIC POLYPECTOMY removal of a colorectal polyp through a colonoscope.

COLONOGRAPHY a CT scan of the colon.

COLOSTOMY the opening created when the anus must be removed and the end of the colon is brought up to an opening in the abdominal wall.

COMPLEMENTARY THERAPY a treatment designed to supplement standard medical practice.

COMBINATION THERAPY treatment consisting of more than one drug at a time.

CT SCAN/CAT SCAN a complex device containing several X-ray machines coordinated by a computer to create what appears to be a "slice" of the body.

DESCENDING COLON the portion of the colon going down the left side of the abdomen.

DIVERTICULITIS inflammation due to a perforation of a diverticulum.

EARLY STAGE a young cancer that has not spread.

EEA an end-to-end anastomosis stapler used to join the intestine in an anterior resection operation

EN BLOC RESECTION an operation in which a group of two or more organs or parts of organs are removed in one piece in order to avoid disturbing a cancer that connects the organs.

ENDORECTAL ULTRASOUND an ultrasound of the anus and rectum as well as surrounding tissues obtained by a special ultrasound probe that is placed into the rectum through the anus.

ENDOSCOPY SUITE a special clinic where colonoscopy and other scope procedures are carried out.

ERYTHROPOEITIN a hormone given to help stimulate bone marrow to produce more red blood cells.

FAMILIAL ADENOMATOUS POLYPOSIS see *FAP*.

FAMILIAL COLORECTAL CANCER see *FCC*.

FAP (familial adenomatous polyposis) a colorectal cancer syndrome inherited at birth, involving multiple colorectal polyps. (It accounts for about 1% of all colorectal cancers.)

FCC (familial colorectal cancer) the term used for the 10% to 15% of patients with colorectal cancer or adenomas who have other affected family members, but do not fit the criteria for FAP or HNPCC.

FECAL OCCULT BLOOD TEST a common test used to identify minute amounts of blood (invisible to the naked eye) in the stool. See *occult bleeding*.

FIVE-YEAR SURVIVAL the term used to indicate likelihood of cure of colorectal cancer.

FLEXIBLE SIGMOIDOSCOPE 60 cm flexible scope used to examine the rectum, sigmoid colon, and descending colon.

G-CSF a hormone that helps bone marrow recover and increases the white blood cell count after it has been lowered by chemotherapy.

GASTROINTESTINAL (GI) TRACT the body's digestive system that begins at the mouth and ends at the anus.

GRAY a unit used for measuring radiation.

HEREDITARY NON-POLYPOSIS COLORECTAL CANCER see *HNPCC*.

HNPCC (hereditary non-polyposis colorectal cancer) a colorectal cancer syndrome inherited at birth, accounting for 3% to 5% of all colorectal cancers. It is also called *Lynch syndrome* and *cancer family syndrome*.

HIGH GRADE CANCER an aggressive (poorly differentiated) cancer.

HYPERPLASTIC POLYP a harmless type of polyp often seen in the rectum.

IN SITU CANCER cancer that is confined within the surface of the affected organ.

INCOMPLETE RESECTION MARGIN the cancerous tissue removed from a patient in which the pathologist finds cancerous cells at the edge. It indicates that there is still cancer remaining in the patient.

INTRAMUCOSAL CARCINOMA see *in situ cancer.*

INVOLVED LYMPH NODE a lymph node containing cancer spread.

IRRITABLE BOWEL SYNDROME a benign disorder of the muscles of the colon characterized by cramps and varying types of bowel movements.

INFLAMMATORY BOWEL DISEASE (IBD) a poorly understood disease of inflammation of the intestine.

INFLAMMATORY POLYP a polyp resulting from inflammation.

JUVENILE POLYPOSIS multiple juvenile (mucus retention) polyps that can occasionally be seen together with premalignant and malignant polyps.

LAPAROSCOPY a method of operating on the abdomen using small incisions and narrow operating instruments.

LAPAROSCOPIC ASSISTED laparoscopy in which a larger incision is made and the surgeon is able to place a hand in the abdomen to assist the laparoscopic procedure.

LARGE INTESTINE see *colon.*

LATE STAGE a cancer that has spread significantly.

LEFT HEMICOLECTOMY removal of the left side of the colon.

LIVER METASTASES cancer spread to the liver.

LOCALIZED TREATMENT removing cancer of the rectum through the anus. It is reserved for very small, superficial cancers and designed to destroy or remove the cancer without the need for major abdominal surgery.

LOCALLY ADVANCED deeply penetrating cancer.

LONG-COURSE PREOPERATIVE THERAPY radiotherapy or chemotherapy given to shrink a rectal cancer to make it easier to surgically remove.

LOW GRADE CANCER a cancer that looks unaggressive (well-differentiated) under the microscope.

LYMPHATIC SYSTEM a system of vessels and lymph nodes and organs that collects body fluids and fights foreign substances.

LYMPH NODES small collections of tissue located along lymph channels. Cancer cells may leave the main body of cancer and drift into the lymphatic vessels and float with the lymphatic fluid to the lymph nodes, where they may implant and begin to grow (called *lymph node metastasis*).

LYMPHOID POLYP a type of polyp containing lymphatic cells, usually benign.

LYNCH SYNDROME see *HNPCC*.

MALIGNANT GROWTH a mass of cells that aggressively grows and divides without regard for the needs and limitations of the body. It is more commonly called *cancer*.

MESORECTAL FASCIA a thin membrane that contains the rectum, mesorectum, and lymph nodes.

MESORECTUM consists of the fat surrounding the back and sides of the rectum and the lymphatic vessels and lymph nodes.

METASTASES cancerous cells that spread from their original location to other parts of the body. The words *metastasis, metastatic, metastasize* all relate to this process of disease spread.

METASTATIC CANCER cancer that is growing somewhere separate from the original (primary) cancer—see *secondary cancer*.

MODERATELY DIFFERENTIATED average grade cancer as viewed under the microscope.

MRI SCAN/MR SCAN a sophisticated device that uses magnetic radiation to produce a picture of the inside of the body.

MUCOSA lining of the colon and rectum.

MUSCULARIS MUCOSA a very thin sheet of muscle cells under the mucosa.

MUSCULARIS PROPRIA the thick muscle wall of the colon and rectum.

MUTATION an alteration in a gene that causes the gene to function abnormally.

NASOGASTRIC TUBE a soft plastic tube passed through the nose and down into the stomach. Used to drain fluid and gas from the stomach when the bowel is obstructed.

NEOADJUVANT THERAPY Chemotherapy or radiation therapy given prior to surgery to enhance cure.

OCCULT BLEEDING small amounts of blood from polyps and cancers that cannot be seen by the naked eye. See *fecal occult blood test*.

ONCOLOGIST a physician who specializes in the management of cancer.

OSTOMATE a person with a stoma.

OSTOMY see *stoma*.

PALLIATE, PALLIATIVE treatment or care given to relieve symptoms in a patient whose disease is incurable.

PATHOLOGIST a doctor who specializes in the structure and function of cells and tissues of the body, and who studies how the various changes relate to specific diseases.

PLATELETS blood cells that help in the blood-clotting process.

PNEUMONIA lung infection.

POLYP a growth, often on a stalk arising from a mucous membranes, such as the colon, nose, or cervix. It can be benign or cancerous.

POORLY DIFFERENTIATED cancer cells that are aggressive looking under the microscope.

POSITIVE LYMPH NODE a lymph node containing cancer spread.

PRIMARY CANCER the organ or location in which the cancer first began.

PROCTITIS inflammation of the rectum.

PROCTOSCOPY see *rigid sigmoidoscope.*

PROGNOSIS an estimated prediction of the expected course of the disease.

PULMONARY EMBOLI blood clots that travel to the lungs and lodge within the blood vessels in the lungs.

RADIATION THERAPY the use of high-energy rays to kill cancer cells (also called *radiotherapy.*)

RESECT, RESECTION surgical removal of a part of the body.

RADIATION ONCOLOGIST a physician who specializes in using radiation to manage cancer.

RADIATION PROCTITIS inflammation of the rectum caused by radiation.

RECTUM the last 15 to 20 cm of the colon.

RETENTION POLYP a polyp consisting primarily of mucus cells often called a *juvenile polyp.*

RIGHT HEMICOLECTOMY removal of the right side of the colon.

RIGID SIGMOIDOSCOPE a 25 cm long instrument used for inspecting the inside of the rectum.

RISK FACTOR something that increases one's chance of getting cancer.

SCREENING tests done to detect disease in a person who is feeling well and who has no signs of disease.

SECONDARY CANCER a growing collection of cancer cells that originated in another site (also called *metastatic cancer*).

SEROSA the outer membrane on the colon.

SHORT-COURSE PREOPERATIVE THERAPY preoperative radiation or chemotherapy designed to reduce the chance of recurrence of a rectal cancer in the pelvis.

SIGMOID COLECTOMY removal of the sigmoid colon.

SIGMOID COLON an S-shaped portion of colon in the left lower quadrant of the abdomen.

STAGING a procedure involving a variety of tests to determine the extent of the cancer.

STOMA an opening in the abdominal wall where the end of the intestine is sewn to the skin. This word is interchangeable with the word *ostomy.*

STOMA THERAPIST a health care worker who specialized in helping patients manage their stomas. Also called *enterostomal therapist.*

SUBMUCOSA the layer of tissue just below the mucosa.

TOTAL MESORECTAL EXCISION a relatively new procedure in which the entire mesorectum and the surrounding mesorectal fascia are removed intact.

TNM SYSTEM OF STAGING a way of using characteristics of the tumor (T), the lymph nodes (N), and whether there are metastases (M) to identify how far a cancer has spread.

TRANS-ANAL EXCISION removal of a polyp or cancer through the anus. See *localized treatment*.

TRANSVERSE COLECTOMY removal of the transverse colon.

TRANSVERSE COLON the middle portion of the colon that goes across the upper abdomen from right to left.

TUMOR a lump of any kind.

WELL-DIFFERENTIATED a cancer that looks unaggressive under the microscope. Another term for *low grade cancer*.

WHITE BLOOD CELLS specialized cells that recognize and destroy foreign materials in the body such as bacteria, viruses, and unfamiliar or abnormal cells.

VILLOUS ADENOMA a kind of polyp that frequently occurs in the rectum, often flat and broad.

VIRTUAL COLONOSCOPY a CT scan of the colon. Another term for *colonography*.

ADDITIONAL READING

GENERAL INFORMATION

AMERICAN CANCER SOCIETY COLORECTAL CANCER: A THOROUGH AND COMPASSIONATE RESOURCE FOR PATIENTS AND THEIR FAMILIES. Levin, Bernard; American Cancer Society. New York, NY: Villard Books. 1999.

COLON AND RECTAL CANCER: A COMPREHENSIVE GUIDE FOR PATIENTS AND FAMILIES. Johnston, Lorraine. Sebastopol, CA: O'Reilly & Associates, Inc. 2000.

COLORECTAL CANCER. Memorial Sloan-Kettering Cancer Center. New York, NY: Memorial Sloan-Kettering Cancer Center. 1999. *(CD in English)*

100 QUESTIONS AND ANSWERS ABOUT COLORECTAL CANCER. Bub, David S; Rose, Susannah; Wong, W. Douglas. Boston, MA: Jones and Bartlett Publishers. 2003.

UNDERSTANDING COLORECTAL CANCER: GENERAL AND CLINICAL LEVELS. Oncology Interactive Education Series; Jack Digital Productions; Princess Margaret Hospital. Toronto, ON: Jack Digital Productions Inc. 2000. *(CD in English)*

WHAT YOU AND YOUR FAMILY SHOULD KNOW ABOUT YOUR RISK FOR COLON CANCER. Mayo Clinic. Patient and Health Education Centre. Rochester, MN: Mayo Foundation for Medical Education and Research (MFMER) 1998. *(VHS in English)*

BC CANCER AGENCY. (Website) *www.bccancer.bc.ca*

CANADIAN CANCER SOCIETY. (Website) *www.cancer.ca*

CANCER.GOV. (Website)
www.cancer.gov/cancertopics/types/colon-and-rectal

COLORECTAL CANCER ASSOCIATION OF CANADA. (Website)
www.ccac-accc.ca/

FAMILIAL GASTROINTESTINAL CANCER REGISTRY. (Website)
www.mtsinai.on.ca/familialgicancer/

COMPLEMENTARY AND ALTERNATIVE THERAPY

AMERICAN CANCER SOCIETY'S GUIDE TO COMPLEMENTARY AND ALTER-
NATIVE CANCER METHODS. American Cancer Society. Atlanta, GA: American
Cancer Society, 2000.

COMPLEMENTARY CANCER THERAPIES: COMBINING TRADITIONAL AND
ALTERNATIVE APPROACHES FOR THE BEST POSSIBLE OUTCOME.
Labriola, Dan. Roseville, CA: Prima Health, 2000.

COMPLEMENTARY THERAPIES: EMPOWERING THE CANCER PATIENT
(videocassette). Donnelly, Laurie. Woburn, MA: Xenejenex Productions, 1998.

UNCONVENTIONAL CANCER THERAPIES. Vancouver, BC: BC Cancer
Agency, 2000. Available online:
www.bccancer.bc.ca/PPI/UnconventionalTherapies/default.htm

NATIONAL CENTER FOR COMPLEMENTARY AND ALTERNATIVE MEDICINE.
(Website) *http://nccam.nih.gov/*

COPING, RELAXATION, AND SUPPORT

ANATOMY OF HOPE: HOW PEOPLE PREVAIL IN THE FACE OF ILLNESS. Groopman, Jerome E. New York, NY: Random House, 2004.

EMOTIONAL FACTS OF LIFE WITH CANCER: A GUIDE TO COUNSELING AND SUPPORT FOR PATIENTS, FAMILIES AND FRIENDS. Kapusta, Beth. Canadian Association of Psychosocial Oncology, 2003. Available online: *www.capo.ca*

FROM THIS MOMENT ON: A GUIDE FOR THOSE RECENTLY DIAGNOSED WITH CANCER. Cotter, Arlene. New York, NY: Random House. 1999.

HEALTHY EATING

AMERICAN CANCER SOCIETY'S HEALTHY EATING COOKBOOK: A CELEBRATION OF FOOD FRIENDS AND HEALTHY LIVING. 2nd ed. Atlanta, GA: American Cancer Society, 2001.

CANCER SURVIVAL COOKBOOK: 200 QUICK & EASY RECIPES WITH HELPFUL EATING HINTS. Weihofen, Donna L.; Marino, Christina. 2nd ed. Toronto, ON: John Wiley & Sons, Inc., 2002.

DIETITIAN'S CANCER STORY: INFORMATION AND INSPIRATION FOR RECOVERY AND HEALING FROM A 3-TIME CANCER SURVIVOR. Dyer, Diana. 8th ed. Ann Arbor, MI: Swan Press, 2002.

NUTRITION DURING AND AFTER CANCER TREATMENT: A GUIDE FOR INFORMED CHOICES BY CANCER SURVIVORS. American Cancer Society Workgroup on Nutrition and Physical Activity for Cancer Survivors. *CA: A Cancer Journal for Clinicians 2001;51:153-181* Available online: *www.cancer.org/docroot/pub/ content/pub_3_8x_nutrition_during_and_after_cancer_treatment.asp*

STAYING ALIVE: COOKBOOK FOR CANCER FREE LIVING: REAL SURVIVORS—REAL RECIPES—REAL RESULTS. Errey, Sally; Simpson, Trevor. Vancouver, BC: Bellisimo Books, 2003.

WHAT TO EAT WHEN YOU DON'T FEEL LIKE EATING. Haller, James. Hantsport, NS: Lancelot Press Limited, 2002.

AMERICAN INSTITUTE FOR CANCER RESEARCH. (Website) *www.aicr.org/*

HEREDITARY INFORMATION

HEREDITARY CANCER PROGRAM, BC CANCER AGENCY (Website) *www.bccancer.bc.ca*

HEREDITARY COLON CANCER ASSOCIATION (US) (Website) *www.hereditarycc.org*

GENETESTS WEBSITE, a publicly funded medical genetics information resource developed for physicians, other healthcare providers, and researchers, available at no cost to all interested persons. (Website) *www.geneclinics.org*

JOHNS HOPKINS HEREDITARY COLORECTAL CANCER REGISTRY (US) (Website)
www.hopkins-gi.org
➡ Digestive Diseases Library, select Colon & Rectum
➡ Hereditary Colorectal Cancer

OSTOMIES

OSTOMY DIETARY GUIDELINES. Price, Anita L; Allen, Lynda; Broadwell-Jackson, Debra. Plainfield, NJ: Patient Education Press. 1995.

OSTOMY BOOK: LIVING COMFORTABLY WITH COLOSTOMIES, ILEOSTOMIES, AND UROSTOMIES. Mullen, Barbara Dorr; McGinn, Kerry Anne. Palo Alto, CA: Bull Publishing Co. 1992.

MEDLINEPLUS. (Website)
www.nlm.nih.gov/medlineplus/ostomy.html

UNITED OSTOMY ASSOCIATION INC. (Website) *www.uoa.org/*

UNITED OSTOMY ASSOCIATION OF CANADA, INC. (Website)
www.ostomycanada.ca/

PERSONAL STORIES

STEWIE'S STORY. Stewart, Paul. Mississauga, ON: Roche Oncology. 2002. *(VHS in English)*

UNLESS YOU ASK. Wallin, Pamela. Toronto, ON: Body'n Soul Corps & Ame. 2002. *(VHS in English)*

HERE AND NOW: INSPIRING STORIES OF CANCER SURVIVORS. Dorfman, Elena; Adams, Heidi Schultz. New York, NY: Marlowe & Company. 2002.

MORE DETAILED MEDICAL INFORMATION

GASTROINTESTINAL ONCOLOGY. Abbruzzese, James L. Oxford: Oxford University Press. 2004.

GASTROINTESTINAL ONCOLOGY: PRINCIPLES AND PRACTICES. Kelsen, David P. Philadelphia, PA: Lippincott, Williams & Wilkins. 2002.

CANCER OF THE LOWER GASTROINTESTINAL TRACT. Willett, Christopher; American Cancer Society. Hamilton, ON: B.C. Decker Inc. 2001.

locally advanced, 229–230
poorly differentiated (aggressive), 190
primary, 10
prognosis, 221–223
secondary, 10
Cancer family syndrome. *See* Hereditary non-
polyposis colorectal cancer (HNPCC)
Candida (yeast infection), 248
Capecitabine (Xeloda), 237
Carcinoembryonic antigen (CEA) blood test
defined, 92
for diagnosis of recurrence, 310
follow-up examination, 314
rise in levels, 235–236
Carcinoma-in-situ, 104, 106
Carcinomatosis peritoneii, 206–207, 236
Cartilage, as complementary therapy, 362
Case manager
communication skills, 111–114
defined, 109–110
duties, 110–111
and medical files, 112–113
and patient stress reduction, 113
questions on behalf of patient, 111–112, 113
CAT scan. *See* Computerized axial tomography
(CT) scan
Cat's claw (uncaria tomentosa), 367–368
CEA test. *See* Carcinoembryonic antigen (CEA)
blood test
Cecum
cancer, radiotherapy treatment, 256
as common site of colorectal cancer, 38
and gastrointestinal system, 16, 17
Celecoxib (Celebrex), 35
Cesamet (Nabilone), 244
Cesium, radioactive, 120
Chemotherapy
defined, 227
nutrition during, 296–297
postoperative (adjuvant), 231–232, 252–257
and pregnancy, 248–249
preoperative (neoadjuvant), 102, 106,
229–230, 252
side effects, 228, 241, 243–249
treatment comparison of colon and rectal
cancer, 232–233
treatment schedules
colon cancer, 254–257
rectal cancer, 251–254

uses
in absence of surgery, 228
for cancer in lymph nodes, 20
combined with radiotherapy, 228, 229–230,
251–257
in conjunction with surgery, 227
for metastatic cancer, 233–235
in recurrent cancer, 319
Chemotherapy drugs
combinations
FOLFIRI, 240, 257
FOLFOX, 240, 255, 256, 257
IFL, 240
Mayo Regimen, 240–241
use of, 227
by generic name
5-FU, 230, 237–238, 240, 252, 253, 254,
255, 256, 257
capecitabine, 237, 240, 254, 255, 257
FA, 238–239
fluorouracil, 237–238
Folinic acid, 238–239, 240, 252, 253, 254,
255, 256, 257
irinotecan, 238, 240, 254
leucovorin, 238–239, 240
marijuana, 245–246
oxaliplatin, 239–240, 254, 255
raltitrexed, 238
by trade (brand) name
Adrucil, 237–238
Camptosar, 238
Camptothecan-11, 238
Citrovorum, 238–239
CPT-11, 238
Efudex, 237–238
Eloxatin, 239–240
Tomudex, 238
Wellcovorin, 238–239
Xeloda, 237
treatment schedules
colon cancer, 255–257
rectal cancer, 252–254
Children. *See also* Hereditary colorectal cancers
explaining cancer, 268
juvenile polyposis syndrome, 340
Chiropractic therapy, 364
Citrovorum (leucovorin), 238–239

Computerized axial tomography (CT scan), 94, 95, 314, 318
Computerized tomographic (CT) colonography. *See* Virtual colonoscopy (colonography)
Constipation, avoidance, after radiotherapy, 133
COX-2 inhibitor. See Celecoxib (Celebrex)
CPT-11 (irinotecan), 238, 246
Crohn's disease, 24, 32
Cryotherapy, 198, 254, 256
CT scan. *See* Computerized axial tomography (CT scan)

D
Debulking tumor, 206
Decadron (dexamethasone), 244, 245
Delerium tremens (DTs), after surgery, 168
Demerol, for postoperative pain, 164
Denial, of cancer diagnosis, 264, 265
Depression, as sign of colorectal cancer, 81
Descending colon, 16, 17, 38
Dexamethasone (Decadron), 244, 245
Diabetes
    reducing postoperative complications, 180
    review by specialist before surgery, 152
    and surgical complications, 174
    and wound infection, 177
Diarrhea. *See also* Stool
    gradual postoperative improvement, 293
    managing stoma, 353
    managing with diet, 297
    postoperative period, 170
    side effect of chemotherapy, 246–247
    side effect of radiotherapy, 129, 131
Diet. *See also* Nutrition
    and cancer prevention, 33, 34
    coping with nausea, 278
    garlic, as complementary therapy, 365–366
    green tea, as complementary therapy, 366
    Healthy Eating Plan, 295–296, 300
    importance, during cancer treatment, 296
    macrobiotics, 360–361
    managing stoma, 353–354
    postoperative, 166
Dietitians, 300
Differentiation system, of grading cancer, 217
Digital rectal exam (DRE)
    follow-up examination, 200, 314
    procedure, 57
    signs of cancer at primary site, 82

Dimenhydrinate (Gravol), 244, 245
Diphenhydramine (Benadryl), 244
Disbelief, of cancer diagnosis, 264
Diverticulitis (diverticulosis), 23–24
DNA
    of cancer cells, 237–238, 239
    and HNPCC, 335
Doctor. *See* Pathologist; Surgeon
Dryness, of mouth and throat, 247–248
Duodenum, and gastrointestinal system, 15, 16

E
EEA (end-to-end anastomosis) stapler, 147, 149–150
Efudex (fluorouracil), 237–238
Electrocoagulation therapy, 198
Eloxatin (oxaliplatin), 239–240, 247
Emotional effects. *See* Psychological factors
En bloc resection, 202, 232
Endorectal ultrasound, 93, 95, 125
Endoscope, 57, 87, 88. *See also* Colonoscopy; Sigmoidoscopy
Enterostomal therapist, 158, 345
Epo (Epogen), 244
Erythropoeitin, 243–244
Esophagus, and gastrointestinal system, 14, 15
Exercise
    and cancer prevention, 33–34
    complementary therapies, 302
    lack, as colorectal cancer risk factor, 30, 32
    mobility after surgery, 167
    during treatments, 285
Eye dryness, side effect of chemotherapy, 249

F
FA (leucovorin), 238–239
Familial adenomatous polyposis (FAP), 31, 73, 328, 329–332, 338
Familial colorectal cancer (FCC), 327, 338–339
Family history, of colorectal cancer. *See also* Familial adenomatous polyposis (FAP); Familial colorectal cancer (FCC); Hereditary non-polyposis colorectal cancer (HNPCC)
    rare hereditary cancer syndromes, 31–32, 339
    as risk factor, 31
    screening guidelines, 73
FAP (familial adenomatous polyposis). *See* Familial adenomatous polyposis (FAP)

Ultrasound tests, for staging, 93–94, 95
Understaged cancer, 213
Urination. *See also* Bladder
    catheter, 165
    output monitoring after surgery, 165
    problems due to radiotherapy, 132
    stoma, after total pelvic exenteration, 316
Uterus
    recurrence of colorectal cancer, 316
    removal during cancer surgery, 202, 203

V

Vagina. *See also* Sexual activity
    dryness, 133, 134, 248, 287
    inflammation, 132–133
    recurrence of colorectal cancer, 316
    soreness, 248
Vascular invasion, by cancer, 218
Vegetables, and cancer prevention, 34, 45
Vegetarians, and Healthy Eating Plan, 295
Villous adenoma polyp, 49
Virtual colonoscopy (colonography), 63–64, 66, 68, 69
Visitors, after surgery, 169
Vitamins, 34, 298–299
Vomiting
    drugs for, 244–245
    management of, 277–279
    not caused by radiotherapy, 130
    as side effect of chemotherapy, 244–245

W

Waiting list, for surgery, 151–152
Weight
    gain, during treatment, 298
    loss, as sign of colorectal cancer, 81, 82
    management, and cancer prevention, 34
Wellcovorin (leucovorin), 238–239
Working
    after surgery, 170
    during chemotherapy, 250
    with stoma, 352

X

X-rays
    barium enema, 62–63
    chest, as staging test, 93, 95
    computerized axial tomography (CT) scan, 94
Xeloda (capecitabine), 237

Y

Yeast infection, 247
Yoga, 302

Z

Zofran (ondansetron), 244, 245